# A Smart Guide to Veterinary Parasitology

# A Smart Guide to Veterinary Parasitology

Authors
**Bhaskaran Ravi Latha, M.V.Sc., Ph.D.**
Professor and Head

**S.T. Bino Sundar, M.V.Sc.,**
Assistant Professor
Department of Veterinary Parasitology,
Madras Veterinary College, Vepery, Chennai-600 007
Tamil Nadu, India
Tamil Nadu Veterinary and Animal Sciences University,
Madhavaram Milk Colony, Chennai-600 051, Tamil Nadu, India

SSPH

**SATISH SERIAL PUBLISHING HOUSE**
403, Express Tower, Commercial Complex
Azadpur, Delhi-110033 (India)
Phone : 011-27672852, Fax : 91-11-27672046
e-mail : info@satishserial.com, hkjain1975@yahoo.com
Website : www.satishserial.com

*Published by :*

**SATISH SERIAL PUBLISHING HOUSE**
403, Express Tower, Commercial Complex, Azadpur, Delhi-110033 (INDIA)
Phone : 011-27672852 Fax : 91-11-27672046
E-mail : info@satishserial.com, hkjain1975@yahoo.com



ISBN 978-93-85055-70-6



**Typeset at :** Harminder Kharb *for* Laxmi Art Creation # 9811482328

**Printed at :** Salasar Imaging Systems, Delhi-110035

# Preface

Multiple choice questions are a well-established, reliable method of assessing knowledge of students and are widely used in Undergraduate, Post graduate and competitive examinations. Veterinary Parasitology is one of the important subjects in Veterinary Science curriculum. Apart from board examinations, approximately 30% of objective type questions in any competitive examination in Veterinary Science are related to Veterinary Parasitology. In order to study and memorize a highly volatile subject like Veterinary Parasitology, the subject needs to be granulated under various topics or chapters so that reading, memorizing and recalling the same in examinations becomes much easier to students. With this intention, the book entitled "**A Smart Guide to Veterinary Parasitology**" has been prepared. The contents of this book follow the complete syllabus in the subject of Veterinary Parasitology covering General Veterinary Parasitology, Veterinary Helminthology, Veterinary Entomology and Acarology and Veterinary Protozoology based on the Veterinary Council of India regulations. The entire syllabus is covered under various headings in an easy manner so that students find it very easy to read, understand and reproduce the same in their examinations. Illustrations are also given wherever necessary. We hope that the features of the book will enable the students to build confidence in Veterinary Parasitology and help them to prepare well for the examinations. We are thankful to Satish Serial Publishing House, New Delhi for bringing out the book in a nice manner. Suggestions for improvement will be greatly acknowledged.

**Authors**

# Contents

PART-I

# GENERAL VETERINARY PARASITOLOGY AND HELMINTHOLOGY

- **Trematodes**
- **Cestodes**
- **Nematodes**

Chapter 1

# TERMS USED IN GENERAL VETERINARY PARASITOLOGY AND THEIR EXAMPLES

| S.No. | Definition | Example(s) |
|---|---|---|
| 1. | Parasite | Liver fluke – *Fasciola gigantica* |
| 2. | Homospecific or Homogenetic association | *Trichosomoides crassicauda* a rat nematode where 4-5 male nematodes live in the uterus of female |
| | | Flock of sheep |
| | | Pack of dogs |
| 3. | Heterogenetic or Heterospecific association | Cattle and insect (Flies infesting a cow) |
| 4. | Commensalism | Intestinal protozoa |
| | Obligatory Commensal | *Entamoeba gingivalis* in mouth of humans |
| | Facultative Commensal | Vorticella and pond crustaceans |
| 5. | Phoresis | Mallophagan lice attached on to the Hippoboscid flies and transported to another host |
| | | Mites travelling on a beetle |
| 6. | Symbiosis | Termites and their intestinal flagellates |
| 7. | Mutualism | Sea anemone and hermit crab |

| | | |
|---|---|---|
| 8. | Parasitism | *Haemonchus contortus* in sheep |
| 9. | Predation | Spider preying on house flies |
| 10. | Definitive host | Cattle for liver flukes<br>Sheep for *Fasciola gigantica*<br>Dog for *Echinococcus granulosus*<br>Horse for *Habronema muscae*<br>Chicken for *Ascaridia galli* |
| 11. | Intermediate host | |
| | Invertebrate Intermediate host | Snail for Amphistomes |
| | Vertebrate Intermediate host | Pigs for *Taenia solium* |
| 12. | Passive intermediate host | Snails for trematodes |
| 13. | Active intermediate host | *Tabanus sp.* for *Trypanosoma evansi* |
| 14. | Reservoir host | African wild game animals (antelope) acting as reservoir host for human trypanosomes like *Trypanosoma rhodesiense* and *Trypanosoma gambiense* |
| 15. | Convalescent carrier host | Bovines for *Trypanosoma evansi* |
| 16. | Transport host | Earthworm for *Ascaridia galli* |
| 17. | Paratenic host | Garden lizard and chicken for *Spirocerca lupi* |
| 18. | Mechanical vector | *Tabanus* spp. for *Trypanosoma evansi* |
| 19. | Cyclical/Biological vector | *Glossina* spp. for African trypanosomes |
| 20. | Ectoparasite | Flies, Fleas, Ticks, Lice, Mites |
| 21, | Endoparasite | Helminths and Protozoa |
| 22. | Temporary parasite | Larval stages of *Oestrus ovis* and *Gasterophilus equi*, Mosquitoes, Bugs |
| 23. | Permanent parasite | Sheep ked, Lice |
| 24. | Periodic/Intermittent/ Occasional parasite | Biting flies and soft ticks |
| 25. | Incidental parasite | *Ascaris* in sheep and goats<br>*Toxocara vitulorum* in goats |

| | | |
|---|---|---|
| 26. | Accidental parasite | *Musca* spp. larvae causing Myiasis |
| 27. | Ectopic/Erratic/ Aberrent parasite | Liver flukes in lung |
| 28. | Specific parasite | *Dipylidium caninum* for dogs |
| 29. | Facultative parasite | Calliphorine larvae<br>*Naegleria fowleri* causing primary amoebic meningitis in man |
| 30. | Obligatory parasite | Trematodes and Cestodes |
| 31. | Hyperparasite | Hymenopteran insects like *Hunterellus hookeri* and *Ixodiphagus mysorensis* on dipteran flies |
| 32. | Pseudoparasite/Artifacts | Pollen grain, Starch granule, Yeast, Plant fibres |
| 33. | Monogenetic parasite | Ascarids, Amoeba, Trichomonads |
| 34. | Digenetic parasite | Coccidia, *Plasmodium,* Piroplasmids, Trematodes of higher vertebrates |
| 35. | Spurious parasite | *Moniezia* eggs in dog feces after ingestion of *Moniezia* infected sheep, goat and cattle intestines by dogs |
| 36. | Monoxenous/ Homoxenous/Direct life cycle | Eimerian spp. and Strongyle spp., Amoeba, Coccidia |
| 37. | Heteroxenous/Indirect life cycle | Trematodes and Cestodes<br>*Theileria annulata* in cattle |
| 38. | Facultative heteroxenous parasite | *Toxoplasma gondii* |
| 39. | Obligatory heteroxenous parasite | *Sarcocystis cruzi* |
| 40. | Autoheteroxenous parasite | Man for *Taenia solium* |
| 41. | Parthenogenesis/ Virgin birth | *Strongyloides* spp. of nematodes<br>*Haemaphysalis* spp. of ticks |
| 42. | Paedogenesis/Juvenile multiplication | Redia producing cercaria in trematodes |
| 43. | Metagenesis | Schizogony alternating with gametogony and syngamy in *Eimeria spp.* |

| | | |
|---|---|---|
| 44. | Heterogenetic life cycle | *Strongyloides* spp. |
| 45. | Schizogony | *Eimeria* spp., *Plasmodium* spp. |
| 46. | Sporogony | Piroplasm in ticks |
| 47. | Syngamy | Apicomplexan parasites |
| 48. | Holozoic nutrition | Amoeba - Temporary mouth<br>Ciliates - Permanent mouth |
| 49. | Saprozoic nutrition | Parasitic protozoa and cestodes |
| 50. | Histotropic phase | Larval migration in *Toxocara canis* |
| 51. | Hypobiosis | *Haemonchus contortus* and *Ostertagia ostertagi* |
| 52. | Aestivation (summer sleep) | Snails |
| 53. | Congenital/Transuterine/ Transplacental infection | *Toxoplasma gondii* in human<br>*Toxocara canis* in dogs |
| 54. | Prenatal infection | *Toxocara canis* in dogs<br>*Toxocara vitulorum* in calves |
| 55. | Transcolostral / Transmammary infection/ Lactogenic | *Toxocara vitulorum* in calves<br>*Toxocara cati* in cats |
| 56. | Transovarian transmission | Transmission of Babesiosis (*Babesia bigemina*) by *Rhipicephalus* (*Boophilus*) spp. of ticks |
| 57. | Trans stadial transmission | Transmission of Theileriosis (*Theileria annulata)* by *Hyalomma* spp. of ticks |
| 58. | Anthropozoonoses | Cysticercosis and Trichinellosis<br>Cystic echinococcosis (Hydatidosis) |
| 59. | Zooanthroponoses | Amoebiasis<br>*Taenia solium* |
| 60. | Protelean parasitism | Bots of *Oestrus ovis, Gasterophilus equi* & *Hypoderma lineatum* |
| 61. | Stenoxenous parasite | *Echinococcus granulosus* occurring in dog & jackal, *Haematopinus suis* in pigs |
| 62. | Euryxenous parasite | *Dicrocoelium dendriticum* in cattle, sheep, rabbit and deer<br>*Toxoplasma gondii* |

| | | |
|---|---|---|
| 63. | Synanthropic parasite | House flies, Cockroaches that are present or frequent human dwellings |
| 64. | Diurnal parasites (Active during day) | *Musca domestica, Tabanus sp.* |
| 65. | Nocturnal parasites (Active during night) | Anopheline mosquitoes |
| 66. | Crepuscular parasites (Active at twilight, dawn or dusk) | *Culicoides sp.* (Biting midges) |
| 67. | Uninomial nomenclature | *Haemonchus* |
| 68. | Binomial nomenclature | *Fasciola gigantica* |
| 69. | Trinomial nomenclature | *Pediculus humanus captis* |
| 70. | Order | Ascarida, ends in ida |
| 71. | Super family | Ascaroidea, ends in oidea |
| 72. | Family | Ascaridae, ends in idae |
| 73. | Sub family | Ancylostominae, ends in inae |
| 74. | Naming based on host | *Ctenocephalides felis* |
| 75. | Naming based on location | *Schistosoma nasale* |
| 76. | Naming based on locality | *Stephanofilaria assamensis* |
| 77. | Naming based on person | *Leishmania donovani* |
| 78. | Direct life cycle with no stage of parasite existing outside host i.e. in environment | *Tritrichomonas foetus* |
| 79. | Direct life cycle with existence of parasite stage outside host but no development occur in the environment | *Entamoeba histolytica* |
| 80. | Direct life cycle with existence of parasite stage outside host and also development occur in the environment but no free living stages are found in the environment | *Ascaris suum* |

| | | |
|---|---|---|
| 81. | Direct life cycle with existence of parasite stage outside host in which development and also free living stage of parasite occurs in the environment | *Trichostrongylus* spp. |
| 82. | Indirect life cycle with one intermediate host | *Fasciola gigantica* - Trematode<br>*Dipylidium caninum* - Cestode |
| 83. | Indirect life cycle with two intermediate hosts | *Dicrocoelium dendriticum* - Trematode<br>*Diphyllobothrium latum* - Cestode |
| 84. | Autoheteroxenous | Man for *Taenia solium* |
| 85. | Parasite entering host actively via skin/ percutaneous/oral/ nasal mucosa by penetration | L3 – Hook worms<br>Cercaria – Schistosomes |
| 86. | Parasite entering host passively via oral route by ingestion of the infective stage along with food and water/infected intermediate host | Embryonated eggs – *Ascaris suum*<br>L3 – *Strongyle* spp.<br>Metacercaria – Liver flukes, Amphistomes<br>Sporulated oocysts – Coccidia<br>Cysticercoids – Tapeworms<br>Cyst – *Entamoeba* spp. |
| 87. | Parasite entering host passively via oral route by carnivorism or carrion feeding/uncooked/ undercooked meat consumption | Larvae in muscle – *Trichinella spiralis*<br>*Cysticercus* – Bladder worm stage of *Taenia* spp.<br>Tissue cyst – *Toxoplasma gondii* |
| 88. | Parasite entering host passively via oral route by transcolostral/lactogenic/ transmammary route | *Toxocara canis* in dogs<br>*Toxocara vitulorum* in calves |
| 89. | Parasite entering host passively via nasal route by inhalation | Dust mite – *Dermatophagoides* spp. |
| 90. | Parasite entering host passively via skin by contact | *Psoroptes* spp. mites |

| | | |
|---|---|---|
| 91. | Parasite entering host passively via placental circulation (congenital infection) | Infective larvae (L2) of *Toxocara canis* and *Toxocara vitulorum*<br>L3 of *Ancylostoma caninum* |
| 92. | Parasite entering host passively via genital organs by coitus (venereal transmission) | *Tritrichomonas foetus*<br>*Trypanosoma equiperdum* |
| 93. | Parasite entering host passively via inoculative method through skin by bite of infected vector | Microfilaria – Filariasis - Mosquitoes<br>Sporozoite – Babesiosis – Ticks |
| 94. | Parasite entering host passively via biting wound by contamination | Trypomastigote of *Trypanosoma cruzi* and *Trypanosoma theileri* |
| 95. | Parasite that removes tissue fluids | Blood sucking flies<br>Hookworms |
| 96. | Parasite that cause destruction of host tissue which occurs during entry process of parasite | Hookworm larvae<br>Cercaria of Schistosomes |
| 97. | Parasite that cause destruction of host tissue which occurs after they have entered into the body | *Ascaris* larval migration |
| 98. | Parasite that cause destruction of host tissue due to immunological response resulting in necrosis, dermatitis, edema and granuloma formation | *Schistosoma nasale* granuloma<br>*Oesophagostomum columbianum* causing pimply gut |
| 99. | Parasite that cause destruction of host tissue due to secondary bacterial infection | *Fasciola* sp.: *Clostridium oedematiens novyi* causing<br>Black disease in acute fasciolosis in sheep |
| 100. | Parasite that cause mechanical interference by blockage of lymphatic vessels | *Wuchereria bancrofti* in man |

| | | |
|---|---|---|
| 101. | Parasite that cause mechanical interference by blockage of blood vessels | *Strongylus vulgaris* in horse |
| 102. | Parasite that cause mechanical interference by blockage of bile duct | *Fasciola hepatica* in sheep |
| 103. | Parasite that cause mechanical interference by blockage of gastrointestinal tract | *Ascaris, Moniezia* |
| 104. | Parasite causing hypertrophy | Coccidia |
| 105. | Parasite causing hyperplasia | Liver flukes |
| 106. | Parasite causing neoplasia | *Spirocerca lupi* nodules in oesophagus transformed into granuloma and later into sarcoma |
| 107. | Parasite causing metaplasia | *Paragonimus westermanii* the parasite is surrounded by epithelial cells and fibroblast cells in lungs where one type of tissue transforms into another without intervention of embryonic tissue |
| 108. | Parasite that compete with host for nutrients | *Diphyllobothrium latum* compete with host for Vitamin B12 or Cyanocobalamin leading to macrocytic hypochromic anemia (Pernicious anemia) |
| 109. | Parasite that alters cell integrity | Coccidiosis |
| 110. | Parasite that produces specific toxin or its secretion or excretion may cause irritation, allergy, dermatitis and hypersensitivity reactions | Flea bite dermatitis<br>Tick toxicosis<br>Tick paralysis |
| 111. | Parasite that causes secondary complication leading to fibrosis, | *Spirocerca lupi* causing malignant tumor |

| | | |
|---|---|---|
| | cirrhosis, proliferation of epithelium, endothelium and lymphoid tissue/ malignant tumour formation | |
| 112. | Parasite causing pressure atrophy thereby impairing the functions of the organs involved | Hydatid cyst in liver and lungs<br>*Coenurus* cyst in brain of sheep |
| 113. | Parasite causing anaphylactic shock | Rupture of Hydatid cyst |
| 114. | Allergic or Intradermal test for diagnosis of parasitic infections | Casoni's test – Hydatidosis<br>Monte Negro test - Leishmaniasis |
| 115. | Mucous agglutination test | Trichomonosis |
| 116. | Capillary agglutination test | Anaplasmosis and Babesiosis |
| 117. | Indirect Haemagglutination test | Toxoplasmosis |
| 118. | Haemagglutination inhibition test | Leishmaniosis |
| 119. | Indirect fluorescent antibody technique | Theileriosis, Amoebosis |
| 120. | Radio immunoassay, Countercurrent immuno electrophoresis, Latex agglutination test | Hydatidosis |
| 121. | Complement fixation test | Trypanosomosis |
| 122. | ELISA and Dot ELISA | Theileriosis |
| 123. | Precipitation test | Circum oval precipitation and Cercarian Hullen reaction for Schistosomosis |
| 124. | Tricin test | Trichomonosis |
| 125. | Xenodiagnosis | *Trypanosoma cruzi* infection using Reduvid bugs |
| 126. | Animal inoculation test | *Trypanosoma evansi* in equines diagnosed by inoculating suspected blood to rabbit, guinea pig or hamster and after few days of inoculation |

| | | |
|---|---|---|
| | | looking for the parasites in blood of these lab animals |
| 127. | Non specific/ Chemical tests | Formal gel test<br>Stilbamidine test for diagnosis of Trypanosomosis |
| 128. | Control of parasitic disease by avoiding gazing during early morning (dawn) and late evening (dusk) hours | To control Strongyle infections since larvae are available at dawn and dusk |
| 129. | Control of parasitic disease by controlling vector/intermediate host | Trematodes - snail<br>Cestodes - Oribatid mite, ants, house flies, beetles<br>Nematode - Various intermediate hosts, transport hosts, paratenic hosts and vectors |
| 130. | Control of parasitic diseases by vaccination | Lungworm vaccine-DICTOL and DIFIL<br>Theilerioisis vaccine - Rakshavac T |
| 131. | Age related immunity | Older chicks resistant to *Ascaridia galli* infection<br>Pigs less than 4 months old are more susceptible to *Ascaris suum.*<br>Lambs are more susceptible to *Moniezia spp* (tapeworm) and *Trichostrongyles* (round worms).<br>Young animals are more resistant to babesiosis than older cattle (inverse/reverse age resistance) |
| 132. | Species related immunity | Majority of helminths of cattle incapable of infecting sheep and goats |
| 133. | Breed/Genetic constitution related immunity | Rhode island Red and Plymouth Rock chicken resistant to *Ascaridia galli* infection<br>West African humpless cattle (NDama and Mutura) are resistant to trypanosomosis |

| | | |
|---|---|---|
| | | Red Maasai sheep of East Africa is more resistant to *Haemonchus contortus*. Zebu (*Bos indicus*) shows high resistance to *Boophilus* ticks than exotic cattle (*Bos taurus*). |
| | | Humans who inherit the sickle cell anaemia trait possess haemoglobin S (HbS) which confers resistance on humans to malaria |
| | | Sheep with Haemoglobin A show superior resistance to infections with *Haemonchus contortus* and *Ostertagia circumcincta* as compared to sheep with Haemoglobin B. Sheep with Haemoglobin A mount an effective self cure phenomenon than sheep without Haemoglobin A. |
| 134. | Immunity related to nutritional status of host | Poorly nourished animals are more susceptible to parasitic infections |
| | | Vitamin (A, D & B Complex) and iron deficiency may interfere with establishment and maintenance of host resistance to blood sucking parasites. |
| 135. | Innate resistance | Sheep cannot be infected with *Ascarids* |
| 136. | Actively acquired immunity - Artificial | Babesiosis, Anaplasmosis, Coccidiosis |
| 137. | Premunity/Incomplete immunity/Infection immunity/Coinfectious immunity | Coccidiosis, Babesiosis, Anaplasmosis, Theileriosis, Trypanosomosis and Monkey malaria |
| 138. | Concomitant immunity | Hydatidosis (Cystic echinococcosis) Schistosomosis |
| 139. | Sterile/Sterilizing/ Complete immunity | *Plasmodium cynomolghi* causing Monkey malaria |
| | | Cutaneous leishmaniosis in man |
| 140. | Self cure Phenomenon | *Haemonchus contortus* |
| 141. | Crisis | *Ancylostoma caninum* |

| | | |
|---|---|---|
| 142. | Cell mediated immunity | *Theileria annulata*, *Toxoplasma gondii* |
| 143. | Intercalary host | Cat getting infected with *Capillaria hepatica* by predating on infected rat |
| 144. | Parasitoids | Hymenopteran flies on Dipteran flies |
| 145. | Autoinfection | *Enterobius vermicularis* (Human pin worm or Seat worm) |
| 146. | Retrofection/ Retroinfection | *Syphacia obvelata* (Rat pin worm) |
| 147. | Hyperinfection | *Strongyloides sp.* |

□□□

Chapter 2

# Common Name and Scientific Name of Trematodes

| S.No. | Common name | Scientific name |
|---|---|---|
| 1. | Tropical Liver Fluke | *Fasciola gigantica* |
| 2. | Temperate Liver Fluke | *Fasciola hepatica* |
| 3. | Liver fluke of dogs and cats | *Opisthorchis tenuicollis (O.felineus)* |
| 4. | Liver fluke of cats | *Opisthorchis viverrini* |
| 5. | Oriental liver fluke/ Chinese liver fluke | *Clonorchis sinensis* |
| 6. | Lancet Fluke | *Dicrocoelium dendriticum* |
| 7. | Intestinal Fluke/Giant intestinal fluke/Largest fluke | *Fasciolopsis buski* |
| 8. | Lung Fluke | *Paragonimus westermanii* |
| 9. | Oviduct Fluke | *Prosthogonimus ovatus,*<br>*Prosthogonimus pellucidus* |
| 10. | Blood Flukes | Schistosomes |
| 11. | Nasal Blood Fluke | *Schistosoma nasale* |
| 12. | Intestinal Blood Flukes | *Schistosoma spindale*<br>*Schistosoma indicum* |

| | | |
|---|---|---|
| 13. | Conical flukes/Fleshy flukes/Rumen flukes | Amphistomes<br>*Paramphistomum cervi* |
| | | *Cotylophoron cotylophorum* |
| | | *Gastrothylax crumenifer* |
| 14. | Liver amphistome | *Gigantocotyle explanatum* (*Explanatum explanatum*) |

Chapter 3

# Host-Wise List of Trematodes with Organ of Prediliction

| S.No. | Host | Trematode | Organ of predilection |
|---|---|---|---|
| 1. | **Ruminants** | | |
| | Cattle, buffalo, sheep and goat | *Fasciola gigantica* | Liver, bile duct, gall bladder and rarely lungs |
| | Cattle, buffalo, sheep and goat | *Fasciola hepatica* | Liver, bile duct, gall bladder |
| | Cattle, sheep and goat | *Dicrocoelium dendriticum* | Bile duct |
| | Cattle, goat | *Paragonimus westermanii* | Lungs, rarely brain and spinal cord |
| | Cattle, buffalo, sheep and goat | *Paramphistomum cervi* | Rumen |
| | Cattle, buffalo, sheep and goat | *Cotylophoron cotylophorum* | Rumen |
| | Cattle, buffalo, sheep and goat | *Gastrothylax crumenifer* | Rumen |
| | Cattle, buffalo, sheep and goat | *Gigantocotyle explanatum* (*Explanatum explanatum*) | Bile duct and liver |
| | Cattle, buffalo, rare in sheep, goats | *Schistosoma nasale* | Nasal veins |

| | | | |
|---|---|---|---|
| | Cattle, buffalo, sheep and goats | *Schistosoma spindale* | Potal and Mesenteric veins |
| | Cattle, buffalo, sheep and goats | *Schistosoma indicum* | Potal and Mesenteric veins |
| | Cattle, buffalo, sheep and goats | *Ornithobilharzia turkestanicum* | Potal and Mesenteric veins |
| **2.** | **Equines, Elephants and Camels** | | |
| | Donkey and other animals | *Dicrocoelium dendriticum* | Bile duct |
| | Equines and Elephants | *Gastrodiscus secundus* | Caecum and colon |
| | Equines | *Pseudodiscus collinsi* | Caecum and colon |
| | Equines and Camels | *Schistosoma indicum* | Portal and mesenteric veins |
| **3.** | **Dogs and Cats** | | |
| | Dogs and cats | *Opisthorchis tenuicollis* (*Opisthorchis felineus*) | Bile duct, rarely in intestine and pancreatic ducts |
| | Dogs | *Schistosoma incognitum* | Potal vein |
| **4.** | **Pigs** | | |
| | | *Dicrocoelium dendriticum* | Bile duct |
| | | *Fasciolopsis buski* | Small intestine |
| | | *Paragonimus westermanii* | Lungs, rarely brain and spinal cord |
| | | *Opisthorchis tenuicollis* (*Opisthorchis felineus*) | Bile duct, rarely in intestine and pancreatic ducts |
| | | *Gastrodiscoides hominis* | Caecum, colon |
| | | *Schistosoma incognitum* (*Schistosoma suis*) | Portal vein |

| | | | |
|---|---|---|---|
| **5.** | **Birds** | | |
| | Domestic fowls, geese and wild birds | *Prosthogonimus ovatus* | Bursa of Fabricius or oviduct |
| **6.** | **Man** | | |
| | | *Fasciola hepatica* | Liver, bile duct, gall bladder |
| | | *Fasciolopsis buski* | Small intestine |
| | | *Paragonimus westermanii* | Lungs, rarely brain and spinal cord |
| | | *Opisthorchis tenuicollis* (*O.felineus*) | Bile duct, rarely in intestine and pancreatic ducts |
| | | *Gastrodiscoides hominis* | Caecum, colon |

□□□

Chapter 4

# Intermediate Host(s) of Trematodes

| S.No. | Trematode | First Intermediate host | Second Intermediate host |
|---|---|---|---|
| 1. | *Fasciola gigantica* | Aquatic snails *Lymnaea luteola, L. acuminata, L. auricularia* | ------ |
| 2. | *Fasciola hepatica* | Aquatic snails *Lymnaea acuminata, L. truncatula* | ------ |
| 3. | *Dicrocoelium dendriticum* | Land snail - *Macrochlamys cassida* | Ants (black ants) – *Formica fusca* |
| 4. | *Fasciolopsis buski* | *Planorbis* sp. and *Segmentina* sp. snails | ------ |
| 5. | *Paragonimus westermanii* | Amphibious snails – *Melania* sp., *Semisulcospira* sp. | Crustaceans – crabs or cray fish |
| 6. | *Opisthorchis tenuicollis* | *Bithynia* sp. snails | Cyprinid fish |
| 7. | *Prosthogonimus ovatus* | *Gyraulus* sp. snails | Naiads of dragon fly (Nymph) |
| 8. | *Paramphistomum cervi* | *Planorbis, Bulinus* sp. snails | ------ |

| | | | |
|---|---|---|---|
| 9. | *Cotylophoron cotylophorum* | *Indoplanorbis exustus* | ------ |
| 10. | *Gastrothylax crumenifer* | *Gyraulus convexiusculus* | ------ |
| 11. | *Gigantocotyle explanatum (Explanatum explanatum)* | *Indoplanorbis exustus* | ------ |
| 12. | *Gastrodiscus secundus* | *Indoplanorbis exustus* | ------ |
| 13. | *Gastrodiscoides hominis* | Planorbid snail | ------ |
| 14. | *Pseudodiscus collinsi* | *Indoplanorbis exustus* | ------ |
| 15. | *Schistosoma nasale* | *Indoplanorbis exustus* | ------ |
| 16. | *Schistosoma spindale* | *Indoplanorbis exustus* | ------ |
| 17. | *Schistosoma indicum* | *Indoplanorbis exustus* | ------ |
| 18. | *Schistosoma incognitum* | *Lymnaea luteola* | ------ |
| 19. | *Ornithobilharzia turkestanicum* | *Lymnaea acuminata* | ------ |

Chapter 5

# Important Morphological Characters of Trematodes

| S.No. | Morphological character | Trematode |
|---|---|---|
| 1. | • Indistinct shoulders<br>• Intestinal caeca diverticulated both internally and externally | *Fasciola gigantica* |
| 2. | • Distinct (Prominent) shoulders<br>• Intestinal caeca diverticulated only externally | *Fasciola hepatica* |
| 3. | • Oval body without shoulders<br>• Testes are branched and lie in tandem position in the posterior third of the body | *Fasciolopsis buski* |
| 4. | • Lanceolate<br>• Tandem testes<br>• Vitelline glands occupy middle 3rd of the lateral field | *Dicrocoelium dendriticum* |
| 5. | • Thick set ovoid fluke<br>• Spiny cuticle<br>• Ventral sucker present in the middle of the body | *Paragonimus westermanii* |
| 6. | • Small fluke<br>• Translucent body<br>• Testes in posterior half of body<br>• Typically "Y" shaped excretory bladder | *Opisthorchis tenuicollis* |

| | | |
|---|---|---|
| 7. | • Large ventral pouch<br>• Testes are placed side by side<br>• Uterus crosses from one side to the other (right to left) at about middle of the body | *Gastrothylax crumenifer* |
| 8. | • Large sized ventral sucker at posterior end<br>• Testes are lobed and placed diagonally | *Gigantocotyle explanatum (Explanatum explanatum)* |
| 9. | • Smaller ventral pouch<br>• Intestinal caeca extend upto the posterior end of the body<br>• Testis lie dorsoventrally | *Fischoederius elongatus* |
| 10. | • Smaller ventral pouch<br>• Intestinal caeca short only extending upto the middle of the body<br>• Testis lie dorsoventrally | *Fischoederius cobboldi* |
| 11. | • Body is divided into two portions<br>• Anterior portion is globoid or cone shaped<br>• Posterior portion is papillated discoid or saucer shaped<br>• Oral/oesophageal pouches present | *Gastrodiscus secundus* |
| 12. | • Pyriform in outline<br>• Body is divided into two parts<br>• Anterior part is smaller than posterior and without papillae<br>• Oral pouches present<br>• Ventral sucker has prominent deep cleft | *Gastrodiscoides hominis* |
| 13. | • Body tapering anteriorly and rounded posteriorly<br>• Oral pouches present<br>• Intestinal caeca wavy<br>• Testes deeply lobed placed side by side | *Pseudodiscus collinsi* |
| 14. | • Coarse tuberculations on the cuticle | *Schistosoma nasale* |
| 15. | • Smooth cuticle | *Schistosoma spindale* |
| 16. | • Large number of testes (above 60) | *Ornithobilharzia turkestanicum* |

□□□

Chapter 6

# Trematode Eggs and Their Characteristics

| S.No. | Egg | Characteristics |
|---|---|---|
| 1. | *Fasciola* spp. | • Composite egg<br>• The large size, oval shape, yellowish tint.<br>• Indistinct operculum<br>• Contains yolk cells and germ cells |
| 2. | Amphistome | • Oval shape<br>• Colourless (non-tinted nature)<br>• Distinct operculum<br>• Contains yolk and germ cells |
| 3. | *Schistosoma nasale* | • Characteristic palanquin or boomerang shape<br>• Presence of terminal spine<br>• Fully developed miracidium within the egg |
| 4. | *Schistosoma spindale* | • The Napoleon hat shape<br>• Terminal spine present<br>• Well developed miracidium inside |
| 5. | *Schistosoma indicum* | • Oval shape with a terminal spine<br>• Well developed miracidium in the egg |
| 6. | *Schistosoma incognitum (Schistosoma suis)* | • Oval shape with a subterminal spine<br>• Well developed miracidium in the egg |

| 7. | *Paragonimus westermanii* | • Yellow brown<br>• Oval or elongate<br>• Thick shell<br>• Asymmetrical with one end slightly flattened<br>• Operculum at large end |
|---|---|---|

❑❑❑

Chapter 7

# Pathological Lesions / Disease Conditions Caused by Trematodes

| S.No. | Pathological lesion/Disease condition | Causative trematode |
|---|---|---|
| 1. | Traumatic hepatitis/Haemorrhagic tracts in liver/Enlarged liver honey combed with tracts of migrating flukes in sheep | *Fasciola gigantica* *Fasciola hepatica* (Acute) |
| 2. | Black disease in sheep | *Fasciola gigantica* *Fasciola hepatica* (Acute) – A complication caused by the anaerobe *Clostridium oedmatiens novyi* |
| 3. | Fasciolosis/Fluke cirrhosis/Liver rot/ Clay-pipe cirrhosis/Pipe-stem liver/ Pipe-stem fibrosis/Hyperplastic cholangitis/Gall stone formation in Cattle | *Fasciola gigantica* *Fasciola hepatica* (Chronic) |
| 4. | Submandibular edema/Facial edema/ Bottle jaw condition/ Jowl edema/Post necrotic scarring, Ischaemic fibrosis, Peribiliary fibrosis, Monolobular fibrosis, Perisinusoidal fibrosis, Hyperplastic cholangitis in ruminants | *Fasciola gigantica* *Fasciola hepatica* (Chronic) |

| | | |
|---|---|---|
| 5. | Dicrocoeliosis | *Dicrocoelium dendriticum* |
| 6. | Haemorrhagic duodenitis/Gillar/Pitto | Immature amphistomes |
| 7. | Nasal schistosomosis/Snoring disease/ Nasal granuloma/Actinobody/ Pseudotubercle/ Hoeppli's reaction/Phlebitis/Cauliflower like sessile growth in nasal cavity/ Whistling sounds during breathing/ Copious mucopurulent discharge from nostrils in cattle especially working bullocks | *Schistosoma nasale* |
| 8. | Visceral schistosomosis/Intestinal schistosomosis/Acute intestinal syndrome/ Chronic hepatic syndrome with lesions similar to Clay pipe stem fibrosis/Intestinal syndrome/intestine appears greyish, thickened and edematous due to confluence of the egg granulomata and the associated inflammatory changes | *Schistosoma spindale* |
| 9. | Visceral schistosomosis in Cattle, buffalo, sheep, goats, equines and camels | *Schistosoma indicum* |
| 10. | Visceral schistosomosis in Pigs and Dogs | *Schistosoma incognitum (S. suis)* |
| 11. | Cercarial dermatitis/Swimmer's itch/ Clam digger's itch/Rice-paddy itch/ Lakeside disease in human beings | Cercaria of non human schistosomes especially Avian schistosomes like *Austrobilharzia* and *Trichobilharzia* |
| 12. | Tumor formation in liver/ Carcinoma of liver/ Cholangiocarcinoma in dogs and cats | *Opisthorchis tenuicollis* |
| 13. | Laying of shell less leathery or rubbery eggs, drop in egg production, pendulous abdomen and peritonitis in hens/Discharge of cheesy material from cloaca | *Prosthogonimus pellucidus, Prosthogonimus ovatus* |
| 14. | Local inflammation or deep ulcerative lesions in intestine | *Fasciolopsis buski* |

| | | |
|---|---|---|
| 15. | Eosinophilic peritonitis, pleuritis, myositis and multifocal pleural hemorrhages, chronic bronchitis with hyperplasia of bronchiole epithelium and pneumonia, pneumothorax | *Paragonimus westermanii* |

□□□

Chapter 8

# Common Name and Scientific Name of Cestodes

| S.No. | Common name | Scientific name |
|---|---|---|
| 1. | Double pored ruminant tapeworm | *Moniezia expansa* |
| 2. | Dwarf tapeworm of Horse/Perfoliate tapeworm/Unarmed tapeworm/ Lappet tapeworm | *Anoplocephala perfoliata* |
| 3. | Dwarf tapeworm of poultry/Smallest tapeworm of poultry | *Davainea proglottina* |
| 4. | Longest tapeworm of poultry | *Raillietina tetragona* |
| 5. | Double pored poultry tapeworm | *Cotugnia digonopora* |
| 6. | Armed tapeworm of man/Pork tapeworm | *Taenia solium* |
| 7. | Unarmed tapeworm of man/Beef tapeworm | *Taenia saginata* |
| 8. | Double pored dog tapeworm | *Dipylidium caninum* |
| 9. | Dwarf tapeworm of dog | *Echinococcus granulosus* |
| 10. | Broad fish tapeworm of dog/ Russian tapeworm | *Diphyllobothrium latum* |
| 11. | Liver tapeworm | *Stilesia hepatica* |

❑❑❑

Chapter 9

# Host-Wise List of Cestodes with Organ of Prediliction

| S.No. | Host | Cestode | Organ of predilection |
|---|---|---|---|
| 1. | **Ruminants** | | |
| | Cattle, Buffalo, Sheep and Goats | *Moniezia expansa* | Small intestine |
| | Cattle, Buffalo, Sheep and Goats | *Moniezia benedeni* | Small intestine |
| | Cattle, Buffalo, Sheep and Goats | *Avitellina lahorea* | Small intestine |
| | Sheep and Goats | *Stilesia globipunctata* | Small intestine |
| | Sheep and Goats | *Stilesia hepatica* | Bile duct |
| 2. | **Equines and Camels** | | |
| | Camels | *Stilesia globipunctata* | Small intestine |
| | Equines | *Anoplocephala perfoliata* | Small and Large intestine |
| | Equines | *Anoplocephala magna* | Small and Large intestine |
| | Equines | *Paranoplocephala mamillana* | Small intestine |
| 3. | **Birds** | | |
| | Fowls | *Davainea proglottina* | Duodenum |
| | Chicken, pigeon and guinea-fowl | *Raillietina tetragona* | Posterior half of small intestine |

| | | | |
|---|---|---|---|
| | Chicken and turkey | *Raillietina echinobothrida* | Small intestine |
| | Fowls | *Raillietina cesticillus* | Duodenum |
| | Fowls | *Cotugnia digonopora* | Duodenum |
| | Fowls | *Amoebotaenia sphenoides* | Small intestine |
| | Fowls | *Hymenolepis carioca* | Small intestine |
| 4. | **Dogs and Cats** | | |
| | Dogs | *Dipylidium caninum* | Small intestine |
| | Dogs | *Taenia hydatigena* | Small intestine |
| | Dogs | *Taenia gaigeri* | Small intestine |
| | Dogs | *Taenia multiceps* | Small intestine |
| | Dogs | *Echinococcus granulosus* | Small intestine |
| | Dogs and cats | *Diphyllobothrium latum* | Small intestine |
| **5.** | **Man** | *Taenia solium* | Small intestine |
| | | *Taenia saginata* | Small intestine |

❑❑❑

Chapter 10

# Intermediate Host(s) of Cestodes and Their Bladder Worms

Bladder worms or larval stages of cestodes are seen in their intermediate hosts

| S.No. | Cestode | Intermediate host(s) | Bladder worm |
|---|---|---|---|
| 1. | *Moniezia expansa* *Moniezia benedeni* | Oribatid mites (Grass mites) *Galumna* sp, *Scheloribates madrasensis, S. laevigatus* | Cysticercoid |
| 2. | *Avitellina lahorea* | Psocids, book lice, dust lice | Cysticercoid |
| 3. | *Stilesia globipunctata* | Oribatid mites/ Grass mites | Cysticercoid |
| 4. | *Anoplocephala perfoliata* | Oribatid mites/ Grass mites | Cysticercoid |
| 5. | *Anoplocephala magna* | Oribatid mites/ Grass mites | Cysticercoid |
| 6. | *Paranoplocephala mamillana* | Oribatid mites/ Grass mites | Cysticercoid |
| 7. | *Davainea proglottina* | Slugs and Snails | Cysticercoid |
| 8. | *Raillietina tetragona* | Ants - *Tetramorium* and *Pheidole* spp. | Cysticercoid |

| | | | |
|---|---|---|---|
| 9. | *Raillietina echinobothrida* | Ants - *Tetramorium* and *Pheidole* spp. | Cysticercoid |
| 10. | *Raillietina cesticillus* | Beetles - *Dermestes* sp, *Opatroides frater* | Cysticercoid |
| 11. | *Cotugnia digonopora* | *Monomorium floricola* ants | Cysticercoid |
| 12. | *Amoebotaenia sphenoides* | Earthworm | Cysticercoid |
| 13. | *Hymenolepis carioca* | Beetles, *Stomoxys calcitrans* (stable fly) | Cysticercoid |
| 14. | *Taenia solium* | Pig | *Cysticercus cellulosae* |
| 15. | *Taenia saginata* | Cattle | *Cysticercus bovis* |
| 16. | *Taenia hydatigena* | Sheep, Goat, Cattle | *Cysticercus tenuicollis* |
| 17. | *Dipylidium caninum* | *Ctenocephalides canis* (Dog flea), *Heterodoxus spiniger* (Dog louse) and *Trichodectes canis* (Dog louse) | Cysticercoid |
| 18. | *Taenia multiceps* | Sheep | *Coenurus cerebralis* |
| 19. | *Taenia gaigeri* | Goat | *Coenurus gaigeri* |
| 20. | *Echinococcus granulosus* | Herbivores, omnivores, carnivores and man | Hydatid cyst |
| 21. | *Mesocestoides lineatus* | 1. Oribatid mite or Coprophagus beetles<br>2. Amphibia, reptiles, birds, dog and cat | Tetrathyridium |
| 22. | *Taenia taeniformis* | Rodents and Rabbits | Strobilocercus |
| 23. | *Diphyllobothrium latum* | 1. Cyclops - (*Diaptomus gracilis* – copepod crustaecean) | Procercoid |
| | | 2. Fresh water fish (Pike, Trout, Perch) | Plerocercoid |

❑❑❑

Chapter 11

# Important Morphological Characters of Cestodes

| S.No. | Morphological character | Cestode |
|---|---|---|
| **Cestodes of ruminants** | | |
| 1. | Inter-proglottidal glands extending throughout the breadth of the segment along the posterior border | *Moniezia expansa* mature segment |
| 2. | Inter-proglottidal glands linear, band like and restricted to the mid region | *Moniezia benedeni* mature segment |
| 3. | • Scolex-large sized head<br>• Outwardly and forwardly directed suckers | *Avitellina lahorea* |
| 4. | • Single set of genitalia<br>• Irregularly alternate genital openings<br>• Absence of vitelline glands | *Avitellina lahorea* mature segment |
| 5. | Single snail shaped par uterine organ in each segment containing numerous eggs | *Avitellina lahorea* gravid segment |
| 6. | Uterus dumb-bell shaped with two portions united by a transverse duct | *Stilesia globipunctata* mature segment |
| 7. | Double par uterine organs in each segment | *Stilesia globipunctata* gravid segment |
| **Cestodes of equines** | | |
| 8. | • Unarmed scolex<br>• Four lappets behind each sucker | *Anoplocephala perfoliata* |

9. • Scolex is narrow — *Paranoplocephala mamillana*
   • Opening of suckes are slit like
   • Lappets absent

**Cestodes of poultry**

10. • Small tapeworm — *Davainea proglottina*
    • Only 4-9 proglottids
    • Armed scolex and rostellum

11. • Oval suckers — *Raillietina tetragona*
    • Rostellum with hammer shaped hooks

12. • Scolex is heavily armed with the hammer shaped hooks in two rows — *Raillietina echinobothrida*
    • Suckers are circular and armed with 2 rows of hooks

13. Gravid proglottids frequently separate in the middle forming small "windows" in the strobila — *Raillietina echinobothrida*

14. • Large with wide armed rostellum having 400-500 small hooks — *Raillietina cesticillus*
    • Suckers are inconspicuous and unarmed

15. • Small tape worm, less than 4 mm long — *Amoebotaenia sphenoides*
    • Elongate, triangular shape

16. • Rostellum with spanner shaped hooks — *Hymenolepis carioca*
    • Suckers unarmed

**Cestodes of dogs**

17. Scolex with pen knife shaped hooks (handle, a guard and a blade) — *Taenia sp.*

18. • Single bilobed ovary placed posteriorly — *Taenia sp.*
    • Uterus is straight and tubular occupying the middle regions of the segment

19. Rostellum with 3-4 rows of spirally arranged rose-thorn shaped hooks — *Dipylidium caninum*

20. • Two sets of genitalia with bilateral genital pores — *Dipylidium caninum* mature segment

| | | |
|---|---|---|
| | • Ovary appear like bunch of grapes on either side of the mature segments | |
| 21. | Cucumber seed shaped segments with numerous large sized egg packets or capsules, each containing 4-20 eggs | *Dipylidium caninum* gravid segment |
| 22. | • Body consists of only 4 segments<br>• The last one being gravid segment and measuring nearly half the length of the parasite | *Echinococcus granulosus* |
| 23. | Scolex is almond shaped bearing longitudinal shallow grooves called bothrida | *Diphyllobothrium latum* |

**Cestodes of man**

| | | |
|---|---|---|
| 24. | The uterine stem with lateral uterine branches and atrophied nature of other organs | *Taenia solium* gravid segment |

❑❑❑

15. Which of the following is not a drug of choice for treatment of Nasal Schistosomosis

A. Triclabendazole

B. Sodium antimony tartrate

C. Lithium antimony thiomalate

D. Praziquantel

16. In amphistomosis, which of the following stages are highly pathogenic

A. Adult flukes B. Immature flukes

C. Cercaria D. Eggs

17. The only amphistome present in liver and bile duct of ruminants is

A. *Gastrothylax crumenifer*

B. *Cotylophoron cotylophoron*

C. *Gigantocotyle explanatum*

D. *Paramphistomum cervi*

18. "Plug Feeding" is characteristic of

A. Immature Liver flukes B. Immature Amphistomes

C. Adult Liver flukes D. Adult Schistosomes

19. The sporangia of the fungus "*Pilobolus*" is involved in the transmission of

A. Ascarid worms B. Eye worms

C. Lung worms D. Stomach worms

20. Hydatidosis occurs by

A. Accidental ingestion of eggs of *Echinococcus granulosus*

B. Ingestion of fertile hydatid cyst fluid with ulcers in the intestine

C. Spillage of fertile hydatid cyst fluid on cut wounds in hands and fingers during slaughter of infected animals

D. All the above

□□□

Chapter 12

# Cestode Eggs and Their Characteristics

| S.No. | Egg | Characteristics |
|---|---|---|
| 1. | *Moniezia* sp. | Egg shell capsule is roughly square with rounded corners, some may be triangular in shape (*M.expansa* - triangular, *M. benedeni* square).<br>Embryophore is pear shaped and is called pyriform apparatus and may be present or absent.<br>Contains an embryo with 6 hooks (hexacanth embryo, hexa - six; acanthor - hooks). |
| 2. | *Taenia* sp. | The thick shell with radial striations giving a Cart wheel appearance<br>The hexacanth embryo (onchosphere)<br>The yellow tint |
| 3. | *Dipylidium caninum* | Large oval capsules (100-400 by 50-200 µm) containing 4 to 20 eggs which are thick |
| 4. | *Diphyllobothrium latum* | Yellowish brown coloured<br>Small oval egg with thin shell (similar to trematode egg)<br>Ends appear pointed than round<br>Operculum present |

❑❑❑

Chapter 13

# Pathological Lesions/Disease Conditions Caused by Cestodes

| S.No. | Pathological lesion/Disease condition | Causative cestode |
|---|---|---|
| 1. | Partial occlusion of ileo-caecal orifice in horses | *Anoplocephala perfoliata* |
| 2. | Nodule formation in intestine of ruminants | *Stilesia globipunctata* |
| 3. | Ulcerative duodenitis in fowls | *Davainea proglottina* |
| 4. | Nodular taeniasis in fowls | *Raillietina echinobothridia* |
| 5. | Anal pruritus/Dragging of perianal region/Scooting in dogs | *Dipylidium caninum* |
| 6. | Traumatic hepatitis/Hepatitis cysticercosa | *Cysticercus tenuicollis*, the bladder worm of *Taenia hydatigena* |
| 7. | Gid/Sturdy/Staggers/Acute meningoencephalitis in sheep | *Coenurus cerebralis*, the bladder worm of *Taenia multiceps* |
| 8. | Measly pork in pigs | *Cysticercus cellulosae*, the bladder worm of *Taenia solium* |
| 9. | Measly beef in cattle | *Cysticercus bovis*, the bladder worm of *Taenia saginata* |
| 10. | Neurocysticercosis in human beings | *Cysticercus cellulosae*, the bladder worm of *Taenia solium* |

| | | |
|---|---|---|
| | | *Cysticercus racemosus* (cyst which has degenerated or grown unobstructed by surrounding tissue) |
| 11. | Hydatidosis in human beings and warm blooded animals | Hydatid cyst, the bladder worm of *Echinococcus granulosus* |
| 12. | Pernicious anaemia/ Macrocytic hypochromic anemia in man | *Diphyllobothrium latum* |

Chapter 14

# Common Name and Scientific Name of Nematodes

| S.No. | Common name | Scientific name |
|---|---|---|
| 1. | Large roundworm of pig | *Ascaris suum* |
| 2. | Arrow headed worm | *Toxocara canis* |
| 3. | Large intestinal worm of cattle and buffalo | *Toxocara vitulorum* |
| 4. | Large roundworm of poultry | *Ascaridia galli* |
| 5. | Caecal worm of poultry | *Heterakis gallinarum* |
| 6. | Pin worm of horse/False whip worm | *Oxyuris equi* |
| 7. | Thread worm | *Strongyloides papillosus* |
| 8. | Red worm of horses/Blood worm of horses | *Strongylus vulgaris* |
| 9. | Nodular worm of sheep | *Oesophagostomum columbianum* |
| 10. | Nodular worm of cattle | *Oesophagostomum radiatum* |
| 11. | Gape worm of poultry/Red worm of poultry/Forked worm | *Syngamus trachea* |
| 12. | Hook worm of dogs | *Ancylostoma caninum* |
| 13. | Hook worm of cats | *Ancylostoma tubaeforme* |
| 14. | Hook worm of sheep and goats | *Bunostomum trigonocephalum* |

| | | |
|---|---|---|
| 15. | Hook worm of cattle | *Bunostomum phlebotomum* |
| 16. | Kidney worm of swine | *Stephanurus dentatus* |
| 17. | Stomach worm/Barber's pole worm/Wire worm of ruminants | *Haemonchus contortus* |
| 18. | Black scour worm/Hair worm | *Trichostrongylus axei* |
| 19. | Brown stomach worm | *Ostertagia ostertagi* |
| 20. | Lung worm of sheep | *Dictyocaulus filaria* |
| 21. | Lung worm of cattle | *Dictyocaulus viviparus* |
| 22. | Red lung worm of sheep and goats | *Protostrongylus rufescens* |
| 23. | Stomach worm of equines | *Draschia megastoma*, *Habronema muscae* and *Habronema majus* *(H. microstoma)* |
| 24. | Oesophageal worm/Gullet worm of dog/Park worm | *Spirocerca lupi* |
| 25. | Eye worm/Extra ocular worm of cattle | *Thelazia rhodesii* |
| 26. | Eye worm of dog | *Thelazia callipaeda* |
| 27. | Gullet worm/Zig zag worm/Stitch worm of ruminants | *Gongylonema pulchrum* |
| 28. | Peritoneal worm of herbivores/ Intraocular eye worm | *Setaria digitata* |
| 29. | Heart worm of dog | *Dirofilaria immitis* |
| 30. | Guinea worm/Medina worm/ Sepent worm/Dragon worm | *Dracunculus medinensis* |
| 31. | Thorny headed worm of pig | *Macrocanthorhynchus hirudinaceus* |
| 32. | Whip worm of sheep | *Trichuris ovis* |
| 33. | Whip worm of dog | *Trichuris vulpis* |
| 34. | Kidney worm of dog/Giant kidney worm | *Dioctophyma renale* |
| 35. | Garbage worm/Trichina worm | *Trichinella spiralis* |
| 36. | Stomach worm of cat | *Physaloptera praeputialis* |

❑❑❑

Chapter 15

# Host-Wise List of Nematodes with Organ of Prediliction

| S.No. | Host | Nematode | Organ of prediliction |
|---|---|---|---|
| 1. | **Ruminants** | | |
| | Cattle and Buffalo especially calves | *Toxocara vitulorum* | Small intestine |
| | Cattle, Buffalo, Sheep and Goats | *Strongyloides papillosus* | Small intestine |
| | Sheep and Goats | *Chabertia ovina* | Colon |
| | Sheep and Goats | *Oesophagostomum columbianum* | Large intestine |
| | Cattle and buffaloes | *Oesophagostomum radiatum* | Large intestine |
| | Sheep and Goats | *Bunostomum trigonocephalum* | Small intestine |
| | Cattle | *Bunostomum phlebotomum* | Small intestine |
| | Cattle, Buffalo, Sheep and Goats | *Haemonchus contortus* | Abomasum |
| | Cattle, Buffalo, Sheep and Goats | *Mecistocirrus digitatus* | Abomasum |
| | Cattle, Buffalo and Sheep | *Trichostrongylus axei* | Abomasum and anterior duodenum |

| | | |
|---|---|---|
| Sheep | *Cooperia curticei* | Small intestine |
| Cattle | *Ostertagia ostertagi* | Abomasum |
| Sheep | *Ostertagia circumcincta* | Abomasum |
| Sheep, Cattle and other ruminants | *Nematodirus spathiger* | Small intestine |
| Sheep and Goats | *Dictyocaulus filaria* | Larger bronchioles |
| Cattle | *Dictyocaulus viviparus* | Bronchi |
| Sheep and Goats | *Muellerius capillaris* | Lungs |
| Sheep and Goats | *Protostrongylus rufescens* | Lungs |
| Cattle and Buffaloes | *Thelazia rhodesii* | Lachrymal ducts and conjunctival sac of eye |
| Cattle, Buffalo, Sheep and Goats | *Gongylonema pulchrum* | Oesophagus embedded in zigzag fashion in mucosa or submucosa |
| Cattle and Buffaloes | *Setaria digitata* | Peritoneal cavity |
| Cattle | *Parafilaria bovicola* | Subcutaneous tissues |
| Cattle | *Stephanofilaria assamensis* | Skin - hump region |
| Cattle and Buffaloes | *Onchocerca indica* | Subcutaneous tissues especially brisket and hind limbs |
| Cattle | *Onchocerca armillata* | Aorta |
| Cattle | *Onchocerca gibsoni* | Subcutaneous tissue |

2. **Equines and Camels**

| | | |
|---|---|---|
| Horses | *Parascaris equorum* | Small intestine |
| Equines | *Oxyuris equi* | Large intestine |
| Equines | *Strongylus vulgaris*<br>*Strongylus edentatus*<br>*Strongylus equinus* | Large intestine |

| | | | |
|---|---|---|---|
| | Equines | *Trichostrongylus axei* | Stomach |
| | Equines | *Draschia megastoma* | Stomach tumors |
| | Equines | *Habronema muscae* | Stomach |
| | Equines | *Habronema majus* | Stomach |
| 3. | **Birds** | | |
| | Poultry | *Ascaridia galli* | Small intestine |
| | Fowls, Turkeys | *Heterakis gallinarum* | Caecum |
| | Fowls | *Syngamus trachea* | Trachea |
| | Fowls | *Tetrameres mohtedai* | Proventriculus and Gizzard |
| | Fowls | *Capillaria annulata* | Crop and Proventriculus |
| 4. | **Dogs and Cats** | | |
| | Dogs | *Toxocara canis* | Small intestine |
| | Dogs | *Toxascaris leonina* | Small intestine |
| | Cats | *Toxocara cati* | Small intestine |
| | Dogs | *Ancylostoma caninum* | Small intestine |
| | Dogs | *Spirocerca lupi* | Oesophagus, cardiac end of stomach, aorta |
| | Dogs | *Thelazia callipaeda* | Nictitating membrane |
| | Dogs | *Dirofilaria immitis* | Right ventricle of heart and sometimes pulmonary artery |
| | Dogs and other carnivores | *Dioctophyma renale* | Kidney and other organs |
| 5. | **Pigs** | *Ascaris suum* | Small intestine |
| | | *Stephanurus dentatus* | Perirenal fat, pelvis of kidney, ureter and erratic parasites in liver, thoracic organs and spinal cord |

| | | | |
|---|---|---|---|
| | | *Macrocanthorhynchus hirudinaceus* | Small intestine especially jejunum |
| | | *Trichinella spiralis* | Adult worms in large intestine and larvae in striated muscles |
| 6. | **Man** | *Dracunculus medinensis* | Subcutaneous tissues |

□□□

Chapter 16

# Intermediate Host(s)/Vector(s)/ Transport Host(s)/Paratenic Host(s) of Nematodes

| S.No. | Nematode | Intermediate host(s) | Transport host(s) | Vector(s) |
|---|---|---|---|---|
| 1. | *Syngamus trachea* | --- | Earth worms, slugs, snails and several arthropods | --- |
| 2. | *Habronema muscae* *Draschia megastoma* | *Musca domestica* | --- | --- |
| 3. | *Habronema microstoma* *(H. majus)* | *Stomoxys calcitrans* | --- | --- |
| 4. | *Spirocerca lupi* | Coprophagus beetles *(Scarabeus)* | --- | --- |
| | | **Paratenic host** Garden lizards *(Calotes)*, frogs, mice, chicken | --- | --- |
| 5. | *Thelazia rhodesii* | *Musca viscina* | --- | --- |

| | | | | |
|---|---|---|---|---|
| 6. | *Thelazia callipaeda* | Fruit fly (*Phortica variegata*) | --- | --- |
| 7. | *Setaria digitata* | --- | --- | Mosquitoes - *Culex, Anopheles, Aedes* sp |
| 8. | *Dirofilaria immitis* | --- | --- | Mosquitoes - *Culex, Anopheles, Aedes* sp |
| 9. | *Parafilaria bovicola* | *Musca* sp. | --- | --- |
| 10. | *Stephanofilaria assamensis* | *Musca viscina* | --- | --- |
| 11. | *Onchocerca indica* | --- | --- | *Culicoides* sp. & *Simulium* sp. |
| 12. | *Onchocerca volvulus* | --- | --- | *Simulium* sp. |
| 13. | *Onchocerca gibsoni* | --- | --- | *Culicoides* sp. |
| 14. | *Dracunculus medinensis* | Cyclops *Diaptomus gracilis* (copepod crustacean) | --- | --- |
| 15. | *Dioctophyma renale* | *Lumbriculus variegatus* (Annelid) | --- | --- |
| | | **Paratenic host** | | |
| | | Pike, Frog | --- | --- |
| 16. | *Macrocantho-rhynchus hirudinaceus* | Dung Beetles | --- | --- |
| 17. | *Protostrongylus rufescens* | Snail species viz. *Helicella, Theba, Abida, Zebrina, Arianta* | --- | --- |
| 18. | *Mullerius capillaris* | Species of the nude slugs | --- | --- |

| | | | | |
|---|---|---|---|---|
| | | *Limax, Agriolimax and Arion, and* snails *Helix and succina* | | |
| 19. | *Gongylonema pulchrum* | Coprophagous beetles of the genus *Aphodius* and *Blaps* | --- | --- |
| 20. | *Tetrameres mohtedai* | Cockroach and Grasshopper | --- | --- |
| 21. | *Physaloptera praeputialis* | Flour beetles, cockroach and field cricket | --- | --- |
| 22. | *Gnathosoma spinigerum* | • Cyclops (First)<br>• Fresh water fish (Second) | --- | --- |
| 23. | *Capillaria annulata* | Earthworm | --- | --- |
| 24. | *Metastrongylus elongatus* | Earthworm | --- | --- |

Chapter 17

# Important Morphological Characters of Nematodes

| S.No. | Morphological character | Nematode |
|---|---|---|
| 1. | • Wide head with distinct neck and prominent shoulders<br>• Mouth surrounded by three prominent lips | *Ascaris suum* |
| 2. | • Distinct wider head separated by a prominent neck<br>• Three prominent lips | *Parascaris equorum* |
| 3. | • Distinct narrower head<br>• Prominent shoulders<br>• Three prominent lips | *Toxocara vitulorum* |
| 4. | • Prominent cervical alae with coarse striations<br>• It give the appearance of arrow head to the worm | *Toxocara canis* |
| 5. | • Digitiform appendage at the terminal end | *Toxocara canis* male tail end |
| 6. | • Three lips<br>• Club shaped oesophagus<br>• No posterior bulb | *Ascaridia galli* |
| 7. | • Narrow caudal alae<br>• Short thick and sessile papillae<br>• Equal or sub equal and similar spicules | *Ascaridia galli* male tail end |

| | | |
|---|---|---|
| 8. | • Oesophagus possess a distinct posterior bulb containing valvular apparatus<br>• Pedunculated papillae<br>• Unequal and dissimilar spicules | *Heterakis gallinarum* |
| 9. | • **Hour-glass** shaped oesophagus | *Oxyuris equi* head end |
| 10. | • Truncated end<br>• Single pin-like spicule | *Oxyuris equi* tail end |
| 11. | • Long filariform oesophagus | *Strongyloides papillosus* |
| 12. | • Large and deep buccal capsule<br>• External and Internal leaf crowns present<br>• Two **ear shaped dorsal teeth** at the base of the buccal capsule with dorsal gutter | *Strongylus vulgaris* |
| 13. | • Large bell shaped buccal capsule opens anterior-ventrally | *Chabertia ovina* |
| 14. | • Cone shaped mouth collar<br>• External and internal leaf crowns present | *Oesophagostomum columbianum* |
| 15. | • Absence of external leaf crown<br>• Prominent rounded mouth collar<br>• Well developed cephalic vesicle constricted behind its middle | *Oesophagostomum radiatum* |
| 16. | • Blood red worms<br>• Male and female found in permanent copulation which is typically **"Y"** shaped<br>• Cup shaped buccal capsule | *Syngamus trachea* |
| 17. | • Three pairs of well developed ventral teeth at the ventral margin of the buccal capsule<br>• A pair of dorsal teeth at the base of the capsule | *Ancylostoma caninum* |
| 18. | • Anterior end is dorsally bent<br>• A pair of well developed buccal capsule with a pair of cutting plates at the ventral margin. | *Bunostomum trigonocephalum* |

| | | |
|---|---|---|
| | • A single well developed dorsal cone with a pair of sub ventral lancets is seen at the base of the buccal capsule | |
| 19. | • A pair of ventral cutting plates at the ventral margin<br>• Buccal capsule has one small dorsal tooth at its base.<br>• Two pairs of sub-ventral lancets | *Bunostomum phlebotomum* |
| 20. | • Cup shaped buccal capsule, thick walled, with 6 teeth at its base<br>• Rim bears a leaf crown of small elements and six internal cuticular thickening (**epaulettes**) | *Stephanurus dentatus* |
| 21. | • Pair of cervical papillae very near the anterior end | *Haemonchus contortus* head end |
| 22. | • Bursa has well developed lateral lobes supported by the long slender rays.<br>• The dorsal lobe is asymmetrical and is supported by **inverted 'Y' shaped dorsal ray** | *Haemonchus contortus* male tail end |
| 23. | • The vulva is covered by a cuticular flap-vulval flap which is large and tongue like (linguiform type) or reduced to a small knob (Knob type) | *Haemonchus contortus* female tail end |
| 24. | • The bursa has well developed lateral lobes like a pair of pincers<br>• Spicules are equal, long and slender and united together to their whole length with membranous expansion of the tips | *Mecistocirrus digitatus* male tail end |
| 25. | • Very slender microscopic worm<br>• Excretory pore situated on a notch at the anterior end | *Trichostrongylus axei* |
| 26. | • Cuticle at the anterior end forms a cephalic swelling | *Cooperia curticei* |
| 27. | • Spicules are equal, stout and dark brown in colour and are "**boot or sock**" shaped | *Dictyocaulus filaria* male tail end |

| | | |
|---|---|---|
| 28. | • Funnel shaped pharynx | *Draschia megastoma* |
| 29. | • Prominent coarse cuticular striations | *Thelazia rhodesii* |
| 30. | • Fine cuticular striations | *Thelazia callipaeda* |
| 31. | • Anterior part of the body bears a number of rounded cuticular cordons arranged in rows on both the sides | *Gongylonema pulchrum* |
| 32. | • Presence of peribuccal ring<br>• Prominent triangular crescent shaped lateral processes | *Setaria digitata* head end |
| 33. | • Tail ends in a simple button (smooth knob)<br>• Two prominent rounded lateral appendages on either side of tail end | *Setaria digitata* tail end |
| 34. | • Presence of cephalic papillae<br>• Vulva situated just behind oesophagus<br>• Muscular and glandular portions of oesophagus without a sharp line of demarcation | *Dirofilaria immitis* head end |
| 35. | • Anterior portion is long and slender<br>• Posterior part is short and stout<br>• Male tail end is spirally coiled and has single spicule enclosed in a spiny sheath | *Trichuris sp.* |
| 36. | • Presence of cephalic vesicle<br>• Anterior cuticle has transverse striations<br>• Spicules in males are short and vary with species | *Cooperia sp.* |
| 37. | • Proboscis is globular and is armed with six rows of six recurved hooks each, lies in a proboscis sac.<br>• On either side of the proboscis sac are the elongate hollow organs called **lemnisci** projecting into the body cavity | *Macrocanthorhynchus hirudinaceus* |

□□□

Chapter 18

# Nematode Eggs and Their Characteristics

| S.No. | Egg | Characteristics |
|---|---|---|
| 1. | *Ascaris suum* | Thick shell that is coarsely pitted with prominent bosses or knobs on the outer surface. |
| | | Sub-globular shape, thick shell |
| | | Unsegmented yolk appears as a compact mass in the centre |
| 2. | *Parascaris equorum* | Sub-globular in shape. |
| | | Egg shell is thick |
| | | Unsegmented yolk as a compact mass in the centre. |
| | | The tinted nature of the eggs |
| 3. | *Toxocara vitulorum* | Round or sub-globular in shape |
| | | Unsegmented yolk appears as a compact mass in the centre |
| 4. | *Toxocara canis* | Sub-globular in shape. |
| | | Unsegmented yolk appears as a compact mass in the centre |
| 5. | *Toxascaris leonina* | Sub-globular in shape |
| | | Unsegmented yolk appears as a compact mass in the centre |

| | | |
|---|---|---|
| 6. | *Ascaridia galli* | Oval shape.<br>Thick and smooth egg shell<br>Unsegmented yolk |
| 7. | *Oxyuris equi* | An elongate, oval shape.<br>Flattened on one side.<br>A plug or operculum at one pole |
| 8. | *Strongyloides spp* | The comparatively small size and oval shape.<br>A thin shell with both poles blunt.<br>Well developed embryo (larvae) inside |
| 9. | *Strongyle spp.* | Oval shape<br>Thin egg shell.<br>Segmented yolk. |
| 10. | *Ancylostoma caninum* | Medium size, oval shape<br>Thin shell<br>Segmented (about 8) yolk |
| 11. | *Spirocerca lupi* | Thick shelled and gelatin capsule shaped.<br>Comparatively very small in size.<br>Contains fully developed first stage larva inside |
| 12. | *Trichuris sp.* | Barrel shaped<br>Brownish colour<br>Plug on either end |
| 13. | Acanthocephala | Eggs contain larva called "Acanthor"<br>Eggs are covered with three layers<br>Oval shaped |

□□□

Chapter **19**

# Pathological Lesions/ Disease Conditions Caused by Nematodes

| S.No. | Pathological lesion/ Disease condition(s) | Causative namatode |
|---|---|---|
| 1. | Milk spot liver in pigs | *Ascaris suum* |
| 2. | Thumps/Piglet anaemia | *Ascaris suum* |
| 3. | Colic<br>Pot belly<br>Passing mud or clay coloured foul/ evil smelling dung in calves | *Toxocara vitulorum* |
| 4. | Intestinal obstruction due to worms ball up | *Parascaris equorum* |
| 5. | Pot belly appearance/Tucked up Abdomen<br>Vomiting and mucoid diarrhoea in pups | *Toxocara canis* |
| 6. | Visceral larval migrans (VLM) or Ocular larval migrans in children | Larvae of *Toxocara canis, Toxocara cati, Toxascaris leonina* |
| 7. | Intestinal obstruction in chicken<br>Presence of viable or calficied worms in the albumin part of hens egg | *Ascaridia galli* |
| 8. | Anal Pruritus in horse<br>Rat tailed appearance of tail of horse | *Oxyuris equi* |

| | | |
|---|---|---|
| | Rubbing of base of tail on to hard objects | |
| 9. | Aneurysm of cranial mesenteric artery with thrombus formation or endarteritis<br>Colic<br>Occlusion of coronary artery or brachio cephalic trunk<br>Temporary lameness<br>Passive congestion of testicles in horses | *Strongylus vulgaris* |
| 10. | In horses large number of haemorrhagic ulcers in the intestine<br>Oedematous swelling on the abdomen and leg | *Strongylus vulgaris* |
| 11. | Gapes in chicken | *Syngamus trachea* |
| 12. | Severe anemia<br>Pale mucous membrane<br>Diarrhoea with bloody mucous and passing tarry red coloured faeces in pups | *Ancylostoma caninum* |
| 13. | Cutaneous larval migrans in man (CLM) | Larvae of *Ancylostoma caninum, Ancylostoma braziliense, Ancylostoma duodenale, Necator americanus, Bunostomum trigonocephalum and Gnathosoma spinigerum* |
| 14. | "Ring worm lesion" in gastric mucosa of calves | *Trichostrongylus axei* |
| 15. | Black scours<br>Protein losing gastropathy | *Trichostrongylus axei* |
| 16. | Haemorrhagic gastritis<br>Swollen abomasal mucosa and red bite marks<br>Hyperplastic gastritis in chronic cases in ruminants | *Haemonchus contortus* (Sheep and Goat)<br>*Haemonchus placei* (Cattle) |
| 17. | Abomasal mucosa with nodules resembling Morocco leather | *Ostertagia ostertagi* |

| | | |
|---|---|---|
| 18. | Pimply gut/Knotty gut in sheep | *Oesophagostomum columbianum* |
| 19. | Pimply gut/Knotty gut in cattle | *Oesophagostomum radiatum* |
| 20. | Husk/Hoose/Parasitic catarrhal bronchitis/Verminous bronchitis/ Atelectasis of lungs in ruminants | *Dictyocaulus filaria* (Sheep)<br>*Dictyocaulus viviparus* (Cattle) |
| 21. | Stomach tumor/Summer sore/ Bursati/Granular dermatitis/ Granular conjunctivitis/Cutaneous habronemiasis/ Swamp cancer in horse | *Draschia megastoma* |
| 22. | Cloudy cornea<br>Marked lacrimation<br>Affected eye is swollen and covered with exudates and pus<br>Keratitis and Opthalmia | *Thelazia rhodesii* (Cattle)<br>*Thelazia callipaeda* (Dog) |
| 23. | Oesophageal tumour or nodules<br>Fibrosarcoma/Osteosarcoma<br>Scarring of thoracic aorta<br>Hypertrophic pulmonary<br>Osteoarthropathy<br>Spondylitis<br>Pleuritis<br>Pyaemic nephritis<br>Aplastic anemia in dogs | *Spirocerca lupi* |
| 24. | Papules or blisters in legs turning into ulcer and worm coming out of the lesion in human beings | *Dracunculus medinensis* |
| 25. | Congestive heart failure<br>Pulmonary hypertension<br>Liver failure<br>Soft cough/Haemoptysis in dogs | *Dirofilaria immitis* |
| 26. | Enzootic Cerebrospinal nematodiasis<br>Kumri<br>Lumbar paralysis in horses, sheep and goats | *Setaria digitata* (Immature forms in CNS) |
| 27. | Haemorrhagic nodules<br>Haemorrhagic filariosis | *Parafilaria bovicola* |

| | | |
|---|---|---|
| | Summer bleeding<br>Verminous haemorrhagic dermatitis in cattle | |
| 28. | Worm nest/Wahi/Kasen | *Onchocerca indica* |
| 29. | Hump Sore<br>Chronic dermatitis<br>Verminous dermatitis<br>Cascado in cattle | *Stephanofilaria assamensis* |
| 30. | Ear Sore in buffaloes | *Stephanofilaria zaheeri* |
| 31. | Onchocerciasis in human/<br>River blindness | *Onchocerca volvulus* |
| 32. | Fistulous withers | *Onchocerca cervicalis* |
| 33. | Raw pork disease | *Trichinella spiralis* |

□□□

Chapter 20

# Anthelmintics

**Trematodes**

**Fasciolosis**

| S.No. | Anthelmintic | Dose | Route |
|---|---|---|---|
| 1. | Triclabendazole | 10 mg/kg | Oral |
| 2. | Oxyclozanide | 10-15 mg/kg | Oral |
| 3. | Closantel | 10-15 mg/kg | Oral |
| 4. | Rafoxanide | 7.5 mg/kg | Oral |
| 5. | Nitroxynil | 10 mg/kg | S/C |

**Amphistomosis**

| S.No. | Anthelmintic | Dose | Route |
|---|---|---|---|
| 1. | Oxyclozanide | 15 mg/kg (single or two doses) | Oral |
| 2. | Niclosamide | 100 mg/kg | Oral |
| 3. | Niclofolan | 6 mg/kg | Oral |
| 4. | Resorantel | 65 mg/kg | Oral |

**Schistosomosis**

| S.No. | Anthelmintic | Dose | Route |
|---|---|---|---|
| 1. | Anthiomaline | 20 ml followed by 10 ml for 3 consecutive days | I/M |
| 2. | Praziquantel | 60 mg/kg or 20 mg/kg 3 doses of 4 hours apart | Oral |

**Cestodes**

**Ruminants**

| S.No. | Anthelmintic | Dose | Route |
|---|---|---|---|
| 1. | Niclosamide | 100 mg/kg | Oral |
| 2. | Praziquantel | 10-15 mg/kg | Oral |

**Dogs**

| S.No. | Anthelmintic | Dose | Route |
|---|---|---|---|
| 1. | Praziquantel | 5 mg/kg | Oral |
| 2. | Niclosamide | 100-150 mg/kg | Oral |
| 3. | Taenil (Herbal) | 4-5 g | Oral |

**Poultry**

| S.No. | Anthelmintic | Dose | Route |
|---|---|---|---|
| 1. | Praziquantel | 10 mg/kg | Oral |
| 2. | Niclosamide | 100 mg/kg | Oral |
| 3. | Fenbendazole | 60 mg/kg for 3 days | Oral |
| 4. | Albendazole | 20 mg/kg | Oral |

**Nematodes**

**Ascariasis - Cattle**

| S.No. | Anthelmintic | Dose | Route |
|---|---|---|---|
| 1. | Piperazine compounds | 220 mg/kg at 5 weeks age | Oral |

**Ascariasis - Dog**

| S.No. | Anthelmintic | Dose | Route |
|---|---|---|---|
| 1. | Piperazine compounds | 100-200 mg/kg | Oral |
| 2. | Pyrantel pamoate | 5 mg/kg | Oral |
| 3. | Mebendazole | 10 mg/kg twice daily for 2 days | Oral |
| 4. | Fenbendazole | 100 mg/kg for 2 days, 25 mg / kg b.wt. from 40th day of pregnancy to 2 days after whelping for somatic ascarids | Oral |

**Ascariasis - Poultry**

| S.No. | Anthelmintic | Dose | Route |
|---|---|---|---|
| 1. | Piperazine compounds | 300-440 mg/kg in feed (or) 440 mg/ litre of water for 24 hours | Oral |
| 2. | Levamisole | 1 ml/3 kg body weight in drinking water | Oral |
| 3. | Mebendazole | 30 mg/kg | Oral |

**Broad spectrum anthelmintics - Ruminants**

| S.No. | Anthelmintic | Dose | Route |
|---|---|---|---|
| 1. | Levamisole | 7.5 mg/kg | Oral |
| 2. | Tetramisole | 15 mg/kg | Oral |
| 3. | Mebendazole | 15 mg/kg | Oral |
| 4. | Albendazole | 5-7.5 mg/kg | Oral |
| 5. | Fenbendazole | 5-7.5 mg/kg (Cattle) 5 mg/kg (Sheep and Goat) | Oral |

| | | | |
|---|---|---|---|
| 6. | Oxfendazole | 4.5 mg/kg | Oral |
| 7. | Pyrantel Pamoate | 25 mg/kg | Oral |
| 8. | Morantel tartarate | 10 mg/kg | Oral |
| 9. | Closantel | 10-15 mg/kg | Oral |
| 10. | Febantel | 5-7.5 mg/kg | Oral |
| 11. | Ivermectin | 200 μg/kg | S/C |
| 12. | Doramectin | 200 μg/kg | S/C or I/M |

**Ancylostomosis - Dogs**

| S.No. | Anthelmintic | Dose | Route |
|---|---|---|---|
| 1. | Pyrantel pamoate | 5 mg/kg | Oral |
| 2. | Ivermectin | 200 μg/kg | S/C |
| 3. | Mebendazole | 10 mg/kg (5 doses) | Oral |
| 4. | Fenbendazole | 100 mg/kg (3 days) | Oral |
| 5. | Fenbantel | 10 mg/kg (3 days) | Oral |

□□□

Chapter 21

# Fill Up the Blanks

## General Veterinary Parasitology

1. In case of *Taenia solium* infection, man acts as both definitive as well as intermediate host and this type of life cycle is called as ..............................................
2. Father of taxonomy is ..............................................
3. A parasite having narrow host spectrum is called .................. ............................
4. The period of dormancy or inactivity during summer or hot conditions which occurs commonly in snails is called ............ ..................................
5. A parasite which requires only one host (i.e. definitive host) for completion of their life cycle is called .................................. ............ parasite
6. An invertebrate host especially an arthropod transmitting the infective agent from one vertebrate host to another vertebrate host is called ..............................................
7. .............................................. is a temporary relationship with no metabolic dependence where one organism is passively transported or sheltered by an another organism
8. Association within same genotype is called ............................. ..................

9. ........................................... host harbors a residual parasite in a latent or inactive phase without showing any clinical symptoms
10. Parasite which occurs in a particular species of host or group of host is called .............................................. parasite
11. Disease which is primarily a disease of human beings wherein other animals are getting the infection from man is called ........... ....................................
12. Disease which occur occasionally in which one or few members of the population is affected is called ............................... ...............
13. An obligatory association between two different species in which the organism derive benefits from the host and both host and parasite are benefited by the association is called ................ ...............................
14. ............................................... is an association wherein one organism lives by preying on another organism
15. In ............................................ or ............................................ vector the infective agent is transmitted from one vertebrate host to another vertebrate host in which the infective stage undergoes developmental changes in the vector
16. The carrier host which recovered from clinical disease but remain harboring residual parasites without showing clinical signs is called .............................................
17. In ............................................. the organism derives benefits from the host but the host experiences neither benefit nor harm
18. A host which harbor encapsulated or encysted larval stage of a parasite in the tissues which is infective to definitive host without any further development is called ...............................................
19. Disease or infection naturally transferable between man and animals is called .............................................
20. In ............................................. vector the infective agent is transmitted from one vertebrate host to another vertebrate host in a short time without undergoing any development
21. Parasite which has a wide host spectrum is called .............. ................................

22. Immunity which is associated with clinical cure, complete elimination of parasite and life long specific resistance to subsequent challenges is called ............................................ or ............................................ or ............................................

23. Infection by a parasite which does not produce any clinical signs is called ............................................ whereas infection by a parasite which produces clinical signs is called ................. .............................

24. The carrier host which pick up infection at low level and never suffered at any time due to infection is called ...................... .........................

25. As per ICZN, names of parasites must be .................................. ........... while writing and .................................... while printing

26. ............................................ is the study of principles and practices of classification

27. Association which is commonly called "Living together of dissimilar organisms" is ............................................

28. The transmission of pathogenic organism especially protozoa from one stage to another stage in tick vector is called ................ ..............................

29. When man acquire infection from lower vertebrates, it is termed as ............................................

30. In ............................................ nutrition absorption of nutrients occurs through body surface

31. The temporary cessation of growth of an arthropod where physiological process are stopped or suspended due to environmental factors is called ............................................

32. The non obligatory association between sea anemone and hermit crab in which both organisms benefit is called ................ ..............................

33. A type of immunity which acts against invading larval stage, but not against existing adult parasitic infection is called ............. ..................................

34. The scientific study of diversity of different living organism is called as ............................................

35. .............................................. refers to the scientific study of different zoological organism which affects and parasitize domestic animals

36. A parasite which parasitizes the host for a short period only is called .............................................. or .............................. ................ or .............................................. parasite

37. The obligatory harmful association commonly referred to as "One who eats at another's table" or "One who lives at another's expenses" in which the dependence of organism on its host is a metabolic one is called ..........................................

38. Immunity to superinfection due to the presence of residual parasite is called ..........................................

39. The resting stage during winter which is featured by low metabolic rate is called .............................................. or ..............................................

40. Based on host range, infestation with *Haematopinus suis* in pigs and coccidiosis in chicken are examples for .............................. ............... parasite

41. .............................................. is a congenital infection in which offspring acquire infection from mother through its placental circulation

42. Two breeds of chicken that are resistant to *Ascaridia galli* infection are .......................................... and ..........................................

43. In .............................................. host the infective agent is harbored without any development and the host just transfers the infective agent from place to place

44. Acquired immunity or Induced immunity which is induced by introduction of antigen is ................................. and that induced by inoculation of antibody is called ..........................................

45. Transmission of pathogenic organism from mother to offspring is called ..........................................

46. Two types of passively acquired immunity are ........................... ................... and ..............................................

47. A parasite which parasitizes the host which is not its actual definitive host is called ..........................................

48. Transmission of pathogenic organism through colostrum to the offspring is called .............................................. or ..................... ......................... infection

49. The term "Parasite" is derived from a Greek word .......................... .................... which means ..............................................

50. A parasite which live as a parasite for only a short period is ..............................................

51. The law governing the writing of name of a parasite where scientists have changed its name for valid reasons is known as ..............................................

52. In .............................................. nutrition ingestion of preformed food material occurs through temporary or permanent mouth

53. Poorly nourished animals are .............................................. susceptible to parasitic diseases

54. Parasite which lives on another parasite is called ..................... .........................

55. Association between two organisms belonging to two different genotype is called .............................................. or ....................... .........................

56. Naming of parasites by one, two and three names is called .............................................. , .............................................. and .............................................. , respectively

57. Immunity that is incomplete and can be broken up by large doses or prolonged exposure to organism is called .......................... .................... immunity

58. In .............................................. the parasite multiplies asexually by division of nucleus and cytoplasm and this multiple fission produces large number of daughter cells called merozoites

59. .............................................. is an arrested development of helminthic larvae until favorable conditions for further development

60. The process which occur after fusion of gametes in which sporozoites are formed within the cyst is called .................... ..........................

61. The time period between time of ingestion and onset of clinical signs is called ..............................................

62. .............................................. host harbors sexual stage or mature stage of parasite in which sexual reproduction occur

63. The transmission of parasite through ova or egg of intermediate host or vector is called ..............................................

64. Usually when writing the name of parasites, the generic name should start with .............................................. letter and species name should start with .............................................. letter

65. A smaller organism which live on or in another bigger organism called host depending on it for food and shelter is called ........................... ...................

66. Parasite which lives on the surface of the body is called .............. ............................... and parasite which lives within the body of the host is called ..............................................

67. A natural process that prevents infection, reinfection and superinfection and assist in destruction of parasites and limiting the multiplication of parasites is known as ................................ ..............

68. The process of formation of gametes like micro and macrogametes is called ..............................................

69. The parasite "*Ctenocephalides felis*" is named after .................. ............................. whereas the parasite "*Stephanofilaria assamensis*" is named after ..............................................

70. Life cycle in which the parasite undergoes some developmental changes in the intermediate host before they get transmitted from one host to another host is called .............................................. life cycle

71. The allocation of name for various group of organisms is called as ..............................................

72. Parasitism by juvenile stage of insects in which larvae or bots are parasitic and adult insects are non parasitic is called ...................... .........................

73. Occurrence of disease in more than one continent is called ..............................................

74. The type of immunity in which the host develops immunity during its life time by the introduction of the organism is called .......................................... or ...................................... immunity

75. A vertebrate host which harbors sexually mature parasite of some other species of vertebrate definitive host and acts as the source of infection to actual definitive host is called ........................ ........................

76. ............................................ is an organism which harbors and nourishes the parasite

77. According to ICZN, order ends with ..........................................., superfamily ends with .................................................. and subfamily ends with ..............................................

78. A parasite which is completely adapted for parasitic life only which cannot survive without host is called ............................ ..................

79. The branch of biology which deals with parasites belonging to plant or animal kingdom is called ............................................

80. A parasite which may or may not require more than one host for completion of their life cycle is called .......................................... and a parasite which compulsorily require more than one host for completion of their life cycle is called .............................. ..................

81. An object mistaken for a parasite is called ................................

82. Parasitism caused by endoparasite is termed as ........................... ................... and parasitism caused by ectoparasite is termed as ..............................................

83. Reproduction by young or larval stage of parasite is called ..............................................

84. Life cycle of a parasite in which parthenogenesis alternates with sexual life cycle is called ............................................

85. A disease in which large number of population is affected and the disease spreads very rapidly is called ........................... .................... or ............................................

86. Development of parasite in relation to environment is .............. ..................................

87. The period between the time of ingestion or inoculation of infective agent and it discharges out i.e. demonstration of organism in the feces or blood is called ........................................... or ...............................................

88. The number of parasite that can be harbored by host without manifestation of clinical signs is called ..................................

89. Material to be collected for diagnosis of gastrointestinal helminthic and protozoan infection is ...................................

90. A host which acquires parasitic infection by predating on infected animals is called .............................................

91. The symbiotic association that exist between cattle and egrets is an example for ............................................

92. SNOAPAD stands for ...............................................

93. Immunoglobulin which play a major role in parasitic immunity is ............................................

94. Cells in blood that increase in parasitic infections is ..............................................

95. During the course of evolution, living forms came together and associated as groups to ensure their survival in the environment. This association is referred to as ............................................. or ...............................................

96. Any organism that is intimately associated with another organism of a different species is considered to be a .............................................

97. In parasitism, the organism that derives benefit from the association is called as ............................................. while the other that is harmed is called .............................................

98. .......................... refers to a condition where the juvenile form of a parasite without exiting the host, penetrate in an area adjacent to the site of predilection and establishes in the same host

99. Vector is a latin word which means .......................................

100. ............................................ is the study of disease in relation to the population, aspects of disease such as incidence, transmission and prevalence in a population

101. Parasites generally do not survive below ............................... ................. °C or above ....................................... °C

102. The normal resistance of various species to various pathogens is due to presence of antibodies on their erythrocytes called ........... ....................................

103. ............................................... are antibodies that render the antigens more sensitive for phagocytosis by leukocytes

104. ............................................... are antibodies that inhibit the reproduction of parasites

105. Antigens present on the intestinal surfaces of helminths and arthropods which are not recognized by the host are called ........................................ or ........................................ antigens

## Helminthology

### *Trematodes*

1. Slime balls are seen in the life cycle of ............................................... which contain ...............................................

2. Plug feeding is characteristic of ...............................................

3. Consumption of nuts and tubers of raw water calthrop and water chestnut containing metacercaria could lead to infection with ...............................................

4. Drugs of choice for treatment of *Fasciolopsis buski* infection are ........................................... and ...........................................

5. Fluke of dogs and cats with translucent body, reddish when fresh is ...............................................

6. The name "Helminth" is derived from a Greek word "Helmins" or "Helminthos" which means ...............................................

7. All trematodes are hermaphrodites except ........................... .................... which are unisexual

8. In Phylum Platyhelminthes, the organs are embedded in a specialized connective tissue known as ................................ ................

9. The term "Trematoda" is derived from a Greek word "Treme" which means ...............................................

10. In trematodes, the organ of attachment consists of an anterior sucker known as ............................................. and a ventral sucker known as ............................................

11. Arrangement of flame cells is expressed by a simple formula called Flame cell formula which is useful in ............................................. of species of trematodes

12. In female reproductive system of trematodes, Mehli's and Yolk gland are collectively known as ............................................

13. Hatching of eggs in trematodes is controlled by factors such as ............................................ , ............................................ and ............................................

14. The five larval stages in the life cycle of trematodes in the correct order are ............................................ , ............................... ............... , ............................................ , ........................... .................... and ........................................

15. Larval stage of trematode which is an undifferentiated mass of cells is ............................................

16. In all trematode parasites, the first intermediate host is invariably a ............................................

17. In Schistosomes ............................................ and .................. ........................... larval stages are absent

18. Cercaria of *Dicrocoelium dendriticum* is ............................... .................

19. Egg of *Fasciola* sp. is commonly called ............................... egg and it possess germ cells which are ............................... shape

20. ............................................ form of Fasciolosis is common in sheep whereas ........................................ form is common in cattle

21. Sudden death with bloody discharge from the anus and epistaxis as in the case of anthrax and blood stained froth from nostrils in acute case of a trematode infection in sheep. It is ...................... ........................

22. The three stages in development of nasal granuloma in *Schistosoma nasale* infection are ............................................ , ........................................ and ............................................

23. Flukes which are found attached to the rumen resembling pomegranate seeds are .............................................

24. The amphistome found in liver and bile duct of cattle and buffaloes with a large posterior sucker is .............................................

25. Triclabendazole is the drug of choice for ................................ ...............

26. Control of ............................................. plays a major role in control of all trematode infections

27. Infection by ............................................. fluke occurs in dogs and cats by ingestion of infected raw or undercooked fish

28. Coughing with rusty brown sputum in man is characteristic of infection with .............................................

29. Schistosomes are unisexual flukes in which females are slender and males are stouter and females lie in the ............................... ............... canal of males

30. Eye spots are sense organs found in ............................................. and ............................................. larval stages of liver flukes

31. Fluke infection commonly encountered in temperate regions like Ooty is .............................................

32. Flame cells are also called as .............................................

33. Miracidium hatching out of egg of *Fasciola gigantica* should reach the snail intermediate host within .................................. hours

34. In the life cycle of *Fasciola* each sporocyst gives rise to .................... ......................... rediae by the process called ....................... .......................

35. Under unfavorable conditions, redia will develop into ................. ........................... instead of developing into cercaria

36. ............................................. glands help in formation of metacercaria from cercaria

37. Metacercaria are ............................ in colour with pinhead size

38. Copper sulphate and Baylucide are chemicals used to control .............................................

39. The largest among flukes is .............................................

40. Flukes which are commonly seen as pairs in cysts in lungs are ..............................................

41. Lung worms are very commonly found in the ......................... ..................... lobe of lung

42. A fluke infection in which animals feel thirsty and drink water frequently and additional symptoms with bottle jaw and foetid diarrhea is ..............................................

43. Immature flukes which are pinkish and found in clusters attached to duodenal mucosa are ..............................................

44. As amphistomosis usually occurs along with GI nematode infection, a combination of .............................................. with .............................................. is given to sheep and goats

45. .................................. flukes show marked sexual dimorphism

46. In Schistosomes, eggs are laid in ..............................................

47. Examination of faecal sample taken by rectal pinch is used for diagnosis of ..............................................

48. Hepatic syndrome is an immunological disease resulting from host's cell mediated immune response to eggs of ......................... ...................... in liver

49. Preparation of squash of blood and mucous from faeces is useful in diagnosis of infection with ..............................................

## Cestodes

1. In lambs infection with ........................................ tapeworms predisposes to bacterial infection like Enterotoxaemia caused by *Clostridium perfringens* – Type D

2. The tapeworm which causes deficiency of Vitamin B12 is ..............................................

3. Tapeworm infection acquired by consumption of raw or undercooked infected fish containing pleurocercoid is ..............................................

4. Eating of undercooked or raw pork by human beings will lead to infection with the tapeworm ........................................ which is commonly called ........................................ tapeworm of man

5. Hydatid cyst containing protoscolices is called .......................... ...................... cyst and hydatid cyst which does not contain protoscolices is called ............................................... cyst

6. Tapeworm of man which causes neurocysticercosis is ................. ..............................

7. Ants, slugs, beetles, house flies and earthworms act as intermediate hosts for tapeworms of ........................................

8. Tapeworm found in bile duct of sheep and goats is ............... ...............................................

9. Eating offals with hydatid cyst predisposes dogs to infection with ...............................................

10. The smallest and highly pathogenic tapeworm of poultry is ...............................................

11. Pen knife shaped hooks are found in the rostellum of .................. ............................ tapeworms whereas rose thorn shaped hooks are found in ..............................................

12. Puncture, Aspiration, Injection, Reaspiration technique (PAIR) is used as a method of treatment of ............................................. in human beings

13. The first, second and third larval stages of Cotyloda tapeworms (*Diphyllobothrium latum*) are ............................................... , .......................................... and ...........................................

14. Cooked rice like whitish structures in droppings of birds or dung of ruminants indicate infection with .......................................

15. Consumption of greens contaminated with eggs of *Echinococcus granulosus* will lead to ............................................

16. The term "Cestoda" is derived from a word "Cestus" which means ...............................................

17. In tapeworms, nutrition is by ...................................... method

18. The three parts of a tapeworm are ........................................... , .......................................... and ...........................................

19. In Eucestoda, the hold fast organ or adhesive organ is ......... ............................. whereas in Cotyloda, it is ............................

20. Cup like hold fast organs in Eucestoda are ............................ .................. are groove like hold fast organs in Cotyloda are ...............................................

21. In tapeworms the scolex has a platform like structure known as ...............................................

22. Rostellum which has hooks is called .................................... and rostellum which do not contain hooks is called .......................... ...........................

23. In tapeworms, the body or strobila consists of number of segments called as ..............................................

24. *Railletina* sp. contains .................................... set of genital organs whereas *Cotugnia digonopora* contains ...................................... set of genital organs

25. In Eucestoda, genital pore is situated in .......................... .................... aspect while in Cotyloda genital pore is situated in ............................................... aspect

26. In tapeworms the three types of segments following the head or scolex in the correct order are .........................................., ................................... and ........................................ segments

27. ............................................... tapeworms have separate uterine pore and so they lay eggs singly

28. In tapeworms, the segments packed with eggs is called ............ ................................. segment

29. In Eucestoda the gravid segments are detached and passed in the faeces of the host and the eggs are released due to disintegration of the gravid segment. The process is known as ...............................................

30. In some tapeworms after shedding of eggs, the spent proglottid gets detached and passed in faeces called as .................... ..........................

31. Tapeworm eggs contain six hooked structure called .......... ....................................

32. The four layers in Taenid eggs from outside to inside in the correct order is ........................................ , ............................................ , .......................................... and ...............................................

33. In Cotyloda, eggs hatch out in water releasing a larval stage called ..............................................

34. The larval stages of tapeworms are called ................................ ................

35. ............................................. bladder worm is a single invaginated scolex with cavity filled with fluid

36. ............................................. bladder worm is a single non-invaginated scolex withdrawn into a small vesicle with practically no cavity

37. ............................................. bladder worm is characterized by a single scolex which is not invaginated when fully developed and attached to the bladder by a long neck.

38. ............................................. bladder worm is a large fluid containing cyst in which number of invaginated scolices are attached to the wall

39. ............................................. bladder worm is a large fluid containing cyst which can produce daughter cyst called "Brood capsule" in which scolices develop

40. In hydatid cyst, sometimes the mature brood capsules get detached from the cyst wall and float free in the hydatid cyst fluid called as .............................................

41. ............................................. and ............................................. are the larval stages of Cotyloda tapeworms seen in the first and second intermediate hosts, respectively

42. In Cotyloda, ............................................. larval stage has a solid body and hooks on the posterior region whereas ....................... ....................... larval stage is elongated, solid and has a scolex like that of adults

43. The bladder worm where body is elongate, solid and has a deeply invaginated scolex is called .............................................

44. Tapeworms of Eucestoda need ........................................ number of intermediate host while tapeworms of Cotyloda need .......... ................................ intermediate host

45. *Moniezia expansa* eggs are ............................................. in shape and *Moniezia benedeni* eggs are .................................. in shape

46. *Moniezia sp*. eggs contain oncosphere or hexacanth embryo and has ............................................ apparatus

47. In ........................................ tapeworm, gravid segments are separated by windows in proglottids

48. Tapeworm of poultry which is triangular and elongate is ............. .................................

49. The highly pathogenic tapeworm of poultry is ......................... ....................

50. Vitelline glands and ovary form a mass on either side resembling a bunch of grapes in the dog tapeworm ................................

51. In the gravid segment uterus are replaced by egg capsule or egg packets in the dog tapeworm .............................................

52. Lateral branching of uterus in gravid segments is characteristic of ............................................. tapeworms

53. Bladder worm consisting of a single invaginated scolex, attached to a fluid containing bladder by a long neck commonly found in liver of sheep is ............................................

54. *Coenurus cerebralis* in sheep commonly occurs in ............................ ................. and ................................................ but *Coenurus gaigeri* in goats occur in .............................................

55. In sheep ............................................. bladder worm stages migrate in the brain and spinal cord leaving a tortuous yellowish grey to reddish streaks and it may sometimes also cause pressure atrophy and perforation of skull

56. The most important zoonotic tapeworm of dog is .........................

57. ........................................ dog tapeworm has only 3-4 segments and the penultimate segment is the mature segment and the last one is gravid

58. In hydatid cyst, brood capsules develop from the .......................... .................... membrane

59. Rupture of hydatid cyst leads to ................................................

60. Treating adult dogs with Arecoline hydrobromide to purge out the intestinal contents and to expel all the adult tapeworms is a method to diagnose ................................................

61. Aspiration of cyst fluid, Marsupilization and Sterilization of cyst is the method to treat ..............................................

62. Injection of .............................................. will destroy the germinal membrane and protoscolices in hydatid cyst

63. .............................................. and .............................................. are drugs used to treat hydatidosis

64. Adult *Taenia saginata* tapeworms can grow upto .......................... ...................... meters

65. High density of *Cysticercus bovis* in cattle is seen in ...................... .......................... and ..............................................

66. *Cysticercus cellulosae* in man occurs commonly in ........................ .................. , ...................................... and ....................................

67. In .............................................. tapeworm scolex is unarmed and almond shaped

## Nematodes

1. Larvae of .............................................. are associated with the introduction of the foot rot organism caused by *Bacteroides nodosus* into the skin around the feet of sheep
2. The blood red colored worm which causes nodules in the oesophagus of dogs is ..............................................
3. Pimply gut in sheep is caused by .............................................. and pimply gut in cattle is caused by ..............................................
4. Arrow headed worm of pups causing pot belly is .................. ............................
5. Infection by .............................................. is acquired by dogs due to consumption of paratenic hosts like garden lizards containing encysted larvae
6. The blood feeding nematode causing bottle jaw condition in sheep and goats is ..............................................
7. Zoonotic ascarid infection acquired by children by accidental ingestion of soil contaminated with dog faeces is ........................ or .............................................. and the major ascarid worm involved is ..............................................

8. Severe anemia and passing of tarry red coloured digested blood in puppies is indicative of infection with ..........................................

9. Preventing grazing during dawn and dusk is a managemental method to control .................................................. nematodes

10. Nursing bitches should be properly dewormed to avoid pups getting infected with two important nematodes. They are ................................................ and ................................................

11. GIS which is used for forecasting the occurrence of gastrointestinal parasitic diseases stands for ..........................................

12. McMaster slide is used for ................................................ faecal examination. When eggs are counted using this slide results are termed ................................................ and when oocysts are counted results are indicated as ................................................

13. Modified Knott's test is used to detect ................................................ in blood

14. ................................................ is the endectocide which is contraindicated in "White feet" dog breeds like Whippet, Collie and Australian Shepherd since these dog breeds have a genetic mutation in the multidrug resistance (MDR1) gene

15. Motile larvae (L1) of filarid nematodes found in wet blood film are called as ................................................

16. H11 and HGal GP are vaccine candidate antigens for ..........................................

17. Saturated NaCl used to float helminth eggs is prepared by dissolving ................................................ g of NaCl in 100 ml of water

18. Poultry nematode involved in the transmission of *Histomonas meleagridis* causing black head in turkeys is ................................

19. Round worm depicted in the official symbol of Medicine is ................................................

20. Deworming cattle using Albendazole in early trimester of pregnancy is contraindicated since it will cause ..........................................

21. Nematode in which female worms have reddish blood filled intestines interwining with white uterus or ovaries resembling a Barbers pole is ............................................

22. Apparatus used in culture of non migratory larvae is ................ ..............................

23. ............................................ group of nematodes are commonly called Palisade worms

24. Leaf crowns and Corona radiata are features of ......................... ..................... group of nematodes

25. Large round worm of poultry causing intestinal obstruction in severe infections is ............................................

26. ............................................ is an anemia based chart used to detect *Haemonchosis* in small ruminants

27. ............................................ is the equipment used to detect larvae of *Trichinella spiralis* in muscles

28. Body of nematodes is covered by ............................................

29. Some nematodes have on their cuticle specialized structures such as hooks in ............................................ and cephalic vesicle in ............................................

30. Lateral flat cuticular expansions in nematodes is called ............................................

31. Alae in cervical region is called ............................................ and alae in posterior region is called ............................................

32. Nematodes have a body cavity or coelom but it is not a true body cavity and it is known as ............................................

33. Simple or complicated cuticular thickenings is found in ............................................ nematode

34. Cervical collar or cephalic collar is seen in ........................... .................... nematode

35. The subcuticular layer which forms the cuticle of nematodes is ............................................

36. In ............................................ nematodes, the mouth is surrounded by six lips

37. In Strongyles, secondary structures seen instead of lips are called ..............................................

38. Leaf crown which arises from the rim of the mouth is called .......................................... and leaf crown arising from brim of buccal capsule is called ..............................................

39. Buccal capsule with teeth or cutting plates are features of ..............................................

40. Oesophageal bulb containing valvular apparatus is a characteristic feature of the round worm ..............................

41. Two types of oesophagus in nematodes are .............................. and ..............................................

42. Oesophagus which has a club shaped anterior portion connected by a narrow neck to a pear shaped posterior bulb seen in first stage larva and adult nematodes of non parasitic generation (E.g. Rhabditida) is ..............................................

43. Oesophagus which is club shaped without posterior bulb occurring in second and third larval stages of nematodes and parasitic generation of Rhabditida is ..............................

44. Excretion in nematodes occur by ..............................................

45. Sensory structures which occur as a pair of depression on the head end and tail end of nematodes is called .............................. ............... and .............................................. respectively

46. In nematodes usually male worms are .............................. ................. than females in size

47. Chitinized pigmented structures in male nematodes used for attachment during copulation and to expand the vagina for directing the flow of sperms is called as ..............................

48. In nematodes, cuticular thickening on the dorsal wall of cloaca is called .......................................... and those on ventral wall is called ..............................................

49. Presence of vulval flap or vulval knob in female nematodes is a characteristic of ..............................................

50. Based on the nature of egg laying nematodes are classified into three groups. They are .........................................., .......... .............................. and ..............................................

51. Nematodes that lay eggs containing yolk material when laid as seen in Ascarids are called ..........................................

52. Nematodes that lay eggs containing fully developed larvae as in *Subulura brumpti* are called ..........................................

53. Nematodes that give birth to larvae are called .......................................

54. Mosquitoes are involved in the transmission of ........................... nematodes

55. Eggs of ........................................ have plug at one end whereas eggs of ................................ have plugs at both ends

56. In nematodes the eggs divide and become .................................. and ......................................... stage before larval development is completed

57. In ........................................... nematodes eggs hatch only after ingested by definitive host

58. Example for a nematode where eggs hatch only after ingestion by intermediate host is ..........................................

59. In .......................................... nematodes eggs hatch outside the host in the environment

60. Factors which control hatching of nematode eggs in the environment are .................................. , .............................. , ........................................ and ........................................

61. Important factor controlling the hatching of nematode eggs inside the body of definitive host is ..........................................

62. The process by which the older cuticle of nematodes is replaced by newer one is called ........................ or ..........................

63. Usually nematode larvae undergo .......................................... moults

64. In most of the nematode species third stage larva or L3 is the infective stage whereas in Ascarids the infective stage is ..............................................

65. Examples for nematodes where infective larvae enter into the host though mouth along with feed and water is ................... ....................... and ......................................

66. Examples for nematodes where infective larvae enter into the host though skin penetration is ............................................ and ............................................

67. Examples for nematodes where final host acquire infection by ingestion of infected intermediate host (in pigs) or infective stage injected by intermediate host while feeding (in horses) are ............................ ............... and ............................................

68. Example for viviparous nematode where infection to final host occur by inoculation of infective larvae by vectors like mosquitoes is ............................................

69. A single female Ascarid can lay up to ............................................ eggs per day

70. Tracheal migration or Hepatic tracheal migration is characteristic of ............................................

71. In *Toxocara vitulorum*, in pregnant animals dormant larvae migrate to the mammary glands during .......................... .................. month of pregnancy

72. In calves infection with ............................................ is characterized by diarrhea, steatorrhea, colic and passing of mud coloured evil or foul smelling dung

73. *Toxocara canis* infection is acquired by ................................ , ............................................ , ............................................ and .................................. methods

74. Tracheal route of migration of *Toxocara canis* occurs only in ............................................ and in adults .......................... .................... migration is common

75. In *Toxocara canis* infection, dormant larvae begin to migrate in the pregnant bitches after ............................................ day of pregnancy and enter the foetus

76. In pups acquiring *Toxocara canis* infection through ............. ............................ route, the larvae reach the intestine and directly develop to adults without migration

77. .................................... act as paratenic host for *Toxocara canis*

78. In the life cycle of *Toxocara cati* ............................................ and ............................................ modes of infection are common

79. Nematode which causes inhalation pneumonia and pot belly in puppies is ..............................................

80. .......................................... act as transport host for *Ascaridia galli*

81. .............................................. birds are more susceptible to *Ascaridia galli* infection with respect to age

82. Dietary deficiency of vitamin A, B and $B_{12}$, various minerals and proteins leads to heavy infection with .............................................. ascarid infection in chicken

83. Chicken over 3 months are more resistant to infection with *Ascaridia galli* and this may be accompanied with increase in .............................................. cells in gut mucosa during this age.

84. Large round worm of poultry is ..............................................

85. In chicken viable or calcified .......................................... worms may be found in the albumin part of hens egg

86. In chicken heavy infection with .............................................. ascarid worm cause thickening of caecal mucosa with petecheal haemorrhage on the surface

87. Yellowish white gelatinous streaks of eggs commonly found in perianal region of horses are eggs of ..........................................

88. Scotch tape method is used for diagnosis of infection with .............. ................................ worms

89. Free living and parasitic generation of nematodes is a common feature in ..............................................

90. .............................................. worms have a long filariform oesophagus which occupy upto 1/3 of its length and uterus is intertwined with intestine giving the appearance of twisted thread

91. In *Strongyloides papillosus* infections when environmental conditions are satisfactory, ...................... life cycle predominates and when environmental conditions are unfavourable .............................................. life cycle predominates

92. *Strongyloides sp* which occurs in the small intestine of man, various other primates, dogs, fox is .............................................. and which occurs in birds is ..............................................

93. Worms belonging to Order Strongylida are commonly called ..............................................

94. A median thickening in buccal capsule of Strongyles is known as ..............................................

95. Leaf crowns of .......................................... resemble "palisade" and so they are commonly called as palisade worms

96. Internal leaf crown is also called ..........................................

97. In male Strongyles, the bursa is well developed and bursal lobes are supported by modified caudal papillae known as ..........................................

98. Infective stage larvae of *Strongylus vulgaris* are ............................... ............... geotropic and .......................................... phototropic to mild sunlight, but they will be repelled by strong sun light

99. Infective L3 larvae are found in the grass blades during ................ ........................... and ............................... hours of the day

100. Cervical papillae are characteristic of ..........................................

101. In .................................. worm of sheep the anterior end is curved slightly ventral and the large buccal capsule opens anterio-ventrally

102. .......................................... is a nematode worm which attach themselves firmly to the mucosa of the colon by means of their buccal capsule and draw in a plug of mucosa of the glandular layer and digest the layer by their secretions

103. Transport hosts for *Syngamus trachea* are ................................. .........., .......................................... and ...............................

104. External cuticular thickenings or epaulettes in the leaf crown are seen in ..........................................

105. Anterior end of .......................................... worms are bend in a dorsal direction and they possess well developed buccal capsule and are voracious blood suckers

106. Eggs of *Ancylostoma caninum* are passed in ........................ ...................... cell stage

107. Female *Ancylostoma caninum* lay approximately ...................... ...................... eggs per day

108. In hook worm infections of dogs and cats ............................................ is the common mode of transmission whereas in human beings and cattle the common mode of transmission is ..............................................

109. Four ways of infection in *Ancylostoma caninum* are .................................................... , ............................................. , ............................................. and ..............................................

110. .............................................. worms affecting dogs frequently change the site of attachment and also secrete anticoagulant leading to oozing of blood continuously from the site of attachment in intestine

111. In heavy infection with hookworms puppies becomes anaemic because each worm suck about .............................................. ml per day

112. Type of anemia in hook worm infection of dogs is ...............................................

113. Floor of kennels should be treated with ........................... or .................................. solution to control hookworm infections

114. .............................................. is the hookworm which occurs in the small intestine of the zebu and the ox in India and Sumatra

115. In calves, infection with .............................................. causes *"raised plaque"* like lesion comprises of greyish flat area with sharply demarcated borders looks like *"ring worm lesion"*

116. Each *Haemonchus contortus* worm remove ............................................. ml blood per day

117. .............................................. haemonchosis leads to acute blood loss, haemorrhagic gastritis and dark coloured faeces

118. .............................................. haemonchosis causes anaemia accompanied by hypoproteinaemia and bottle jaw

119. In .............................................. haemonchosis affected animals are weak unthrifty and emaciated causing hyperplastic gastritis and chronic expansion of the bone marrow

120. Abomasum of small ruminants with brownish fluid ingesta and swollen abomasal mucosa with numerous bite marks indictes infection with ..............................................

121. Self cure phenomenon, an immediate type hypersensitivity reaction in haemonchosis is induced by fresh infection with .......................................... in sensitized sheep

122. Largest nematode egg belongs to ..............................................

123. A phenomenon which occurs during late pregnancy and early lactation in animals due to relaxation of immunity and prolactin where hypobiotic larvae become mature to produce eggs is called ..............................................

124. Worms which require intermediate host for completion of their life cycle are called as .......................................... those worms which do not require intermediate host for completion of their life cycle are called as ..............................................

125. In the lungs, .............................................. worms are entangled together giving the appearance of Lumps of broken threads

126. DICTOL/Bovilis Huskvac is a vaccine against .......................... .................... and DIFIL is a vaccine against ............................

127. Widespread interstitial pneumonia in goats is caused by ..............................................

128. Intermediate host of *Metastrongylus elongatus* is ......................

129. Nematode of swine which spreads swine influenza virus is ..............................................

130. Stomach worm of horse which occurs inside tumors is ................ ............................

131. Wart like granular conjunctivitis lesions in horses are caused by deposition of larvae of ..............................................

132. Apart from dogs, *Spirocerca lupi* is also reported in .............. ...............................

133. .............................................. nematode affecting dog is spirally coiled and pink when fresh

134. Common anthelmintics used to treat spirocercosis in dogs are .................................., .................................., ............................. and ..............................................

135. Nematode of birds which shows high degree of sexual dimorphism is ..............................................

136. Stomach worm of cat is ..............................................

137. Ballonets are morphological features in ................................

138. In dogs and cats, young worms of .............................................. migrate through liver causing destruction of liver tissue leaving characteristic "yellow mosaic marking" on the surface and the tracts are filled with necrotic materials

139. The form of second larval stage of filarid worms is called ............... ............................... form

140. In Modified Knotts method for detection of microfilaria, blood is haemolysed by ......................................... and then centrifuged and sediment is stained with ..............................................

141. ............................................... is a commonly used drug for treatment of filarial nematode infections

142. Filarial worms of dogs which is less pathogenic and found in subcutaneous tissue are ............................................... and ..............................................

143. Filarid worm erratically migrating and seen commonly in the anterior chamber of horses and cattle is ..................................

144. Manual removal of worms from skin blisters using a stick by rolling up the worms is a practice to remove ...........................

145. The largest nematode known is ..............................................

146. Mode of nutrition in Acanthocephala is ...................................

147. Eggs of Acanthocephala worms contain the larva called ........... .................................... and female worms of Acanthocephala have a special organ called ...............................................

148. In Acanthocephala, dung beetles ingest eggs which develops into the infective stage called ...............................................

149. Benzimidazoles act by inhibiting the ............................................... and ...............................................

150. Imidothiazoles act by ...............................................

151. Systemic organophosphates act by inhibiting ....................... ........................ enzyme

152. Substituted phenols and salicylanilides act by .........................

153. ............................................. group of endectocides act by potentiating the release and binding of Gamma amino butyric acid in nerve synapses thus blocking GABA mediated transmitters of nerve signals resulting in paralysis of parasites

154. OIE stands for .............................................

155. FAO stands for .............................................

156. WHO stands for .............................................

157. ILRAD stands for ............................................. and is located in .......................

158. BBSRC stands for ............................................. and is located in .............................................

159. ICAR stands for ............................................. and is located in .......................

160. A heritable change in the ability of the individual parasites to survive the recommended therapeutic dose of an anthelmintic is called .............................................

161. *In vivo* tests used to detect anthelmintic resistance are .................. .......................... and .............................................

162. TST stands for .............................................

163. The anemia grade chart based on ocular mucosa colour used to selectively deworm sheep is .............................................

□□□

# Chapter 22

# Multiple Choice Questions

## General Veterinary Parasitology

1. Father of Parasitology is

   A. Carl Linnaeus  B. Aristotle

   C. Francesco Redi  D. Hippocrates

2. A parasite which parasitize an organ which is not its actual habitat or site of predilection is called as

   A. Ectopic parasite  B. Erratic parasite

   C. Aberrant parasite  D. All the above

3. A parasite which can live either as a parasite or free living form is called

   A. Pseudoparasite  B. Obligatory parasite

   C. Hyperparasite  D. Facultative parasite

4. The process in which sexual generation or phase of a parasite is alternating with asexual generation in the life cycle of a parasite is called

   A. Parthenogenesis  B. Paedogenesis

   C. Schizogony  D. Metagenesis

5. Fusion of male and female gametes producing zygote is called
   A. Sporogony B. Syngamy
   C. Merogony D. Gametogony

6. Migration of larval stage of parasite through various organs of definitive host during its development is called
   A. Diapause B. Hypobiosis
   C. Aestivation D. Histotropic phase

7. Reinfection of definitive host by the progeny (ova or larva) of parasite while they are still within the definitive host is called
   A. Congenital infection B. Prenatal infection
   C. Transcolostral infection D. Autoinfection

8. Study of distribution or determination of disease is called
   A. Ecology B. Epidemiology
   C. Demography D. Malacology

9. A parasite which spends a whole life cycle on or in the host is called
   A. Temporary parasite B. Intermittent parasite
   C. Pseudoparasite D. Permanent parasite

10. Some forms of parasite like ova or larva enter into the unnatural host through contaminated water and feed and they are merely passed through the intestine and voided in feces in live or dead form. Such parasite is called
    A. Aberrent parasite B. Hyperparasite
    C. Spurious parasite D. Endoparasite

11. A parasite which require more than one host for completion of their life cycle is called as
    A. Heteroxenous life cycle B. Homoxenous life cycle
    C. Indirect life cycle D. Both A and C

12. Same host acting as both definitive as well as intermediate host is called

    A. Obligatory Heteroxenous    B. Monoxenous

    C. Autoheteroxenous    D. Facultative Heteroxenous

13. The process in which young one is produced without fertilization is called

    A. Paedogenesis    B. Syngamy

    C. Metagenesis    D. Parthenogenesis

14. Occurrence of a particular disease in a particular geographical area at a regular interval that affects a moderate population is called

    A. Sporadic    B. Pandemic

    C. Endemic or Enzootic    D. Epidemic or Epizootic

15. The period between time of ingestion and onset of clinical signs is called

    A. Prepatent period    B. Incubation period

    C. Biological incubation period    D. All the above

16. Immunity to superinfection due to the presence of residual parasite in the host is called

    A. Concomitant immunity    B. Innate immunity

    C. Premunity    D. Sterile immunity

17. The process of establishing and defining different groups of organism is called

    A. Nomenclature    B. Systematics

    C. Taxonomy    D. Classification

18. ICZN stands for

    A. Indian code of Zoological nomenclature

    B. Italian code of Zoological nomenclature

    C. International code of Zoological nomenclature

    D. None of the above

19. According to ICZN Family ends in
    A. "ida" B. "inae"
    C. "oidea" D. "idae"

20. The parasite "*Schistosoma nasale*" is named after
    A. Person B. Location
    C. Locality D. Host

21. The parasite "*Leishmania donovani*" is named after
    A. Person B. Location
    C. Locality D. Host

22. Self cure phenomenon in which adult parasites are expelled due to the super imposing infection of the larvae is a feature in
    A. *Ancylostoma caninum*
    B. *Bunostomum phlebotomum*
    C. *Haemonchus contortus*
    D. *Toxocara vitulorum*

23. Immunity which is genetic or inherited or natural which is not due to previous exposure is called as
    A. Acquired immunity B. Innate immunity
    C. Induced immunity D. Concomitant immunity

24. Immunity in which a particular individual exhibit resistance to a particular organism and even large dose of organism cannot break up the immunity is
    A. Absolute immunity B. Passively acquired immunity
    C. Relative immunity D. Actively acquired immunity

25. Older chicks are resistant to *Ascaridia galli* infection compared to young chicks. This immunity is related to
    A. Genetic constitution B. Age
    C. Nutritional status D. All the above

26. Clinical material to be collected to diagnose nasal schistosomosis is

A. Dung B. Nasal wash
C. Blood D. Skin scraping

27. Method of choice to diagnose mite infestation is

A. Dung B. Nasal wash
C. Blood D. Skin scraping

28. Which of the following is an example of definitive host

A. Mosquito B. Garden lizard
C. Cattle D. Earthworm

29. Which of the following is an example of vector

A. Mosquito B. Garden lizard
C. Cattle D. Earthworm

30. Which of the following is an example of transport host

A. Mosquito B. Garden lizard
C. Cattle D. Earthworm

31. Which of the following is an example of paratenic host

A. Mosquito B. Garden lizard
C. Cattle D. Earthworm

32. In processing of trematodes and cestodes 1% acid alcohol is used as

A. Clearing agent B. Destaining agent
C. Dehydrating agent D. Mounting agent

## Helminthology

1. In trematodes, flame cells are part of

A. Digestive system B. Reproductive system
C. Nervous system D. Excretory system

2. In amphistomes, the acetabulum is

   A. Located at anterior end   B. Located at middle

   C. Located at posterior end   D. Absent

3. Which of the following is not part of male reproductive system of trematodes

   A. Vesiculum seminalis   B. Vas deferens

   C. Receptaculum seminalis   D. Cirrus

4. Which of the following is not part of female reproductive system of trematodes

   A. Laurer's canal   B. Vasa efferentia

   C. Ootype   D. Mehlis gland

5. Eggs hatch only after ingested by snail intermediate host in

   A. *Schistosoma nasale*   B. *Cotylophoron cotylophorum*

   C. *Dicrocoelium dendriticum*   D. *Fasciola gigantica*

6. Larval stage of trematodes which is triangular in shape with ciliated ectoderm which does not feed and penetrate the snail intermediate host is

   A. Sporocyst   B. Metacercaria

   C. Cercaria   D. Miracidium

7. Cercaria of *Fasciola* gigantica is

   A. Xiphidocercous   B. Gymnocephalus

   C. Amphistome   D. Furcocercous

8. The larval form in the life cycle of trematodes which gets encysted in herbage using cystogenous glands and gets ingested by the definitive hosts leading to infection is

   A. Cercaria   B. Redia

   C. Metacercaria   D. Sporocyst

9. In Schistosomes, cercaria enter the host by
   A. Ingestion along with water
   B. Skin penetration
   C. Ingestion along with grass
   D. None of the above

10. Which of the following fluke is lancet or lanceolate in shape commonly found in Himalayan regions and Himachal pradesh
    A. *Schistosoma nasale*
    B. *Cotylophoron cotylophorum*
    C. *Dicrocoelium dendriticum*
    D. *Fasciola gigantica*

11. The optimum temperature for hatching of eggs of *Fasciola gigantica* is
    A. 10°C
    B. 26°C
    C. 5°C
    D. 40°C

12. In *Fasciola gigantica,* infection of snail with one miracidium can produce – – – – – –metacercaria
    A. 100
    B. 50
    C. >600
    D. 10

13. Acute fasciolosis occurs in sheep when the metacercaria ingested is
    A. 500-1500
    B. 2000-10,000
    C. 100
    D. 200-500

14. Nasal granuloma in *Schistosoma nasale* infection is caused by
    A. Adult worms
    B. Schistosomula
    C. Egg containing miracidium
    D. All the above

15. Which of the following is not a drug of choice for treatment of Nasal Schistosomosis

A. Triclabendazole

B. Sodium antimony tartrate

C. Lithium antimony thiomalate

D. Praziquantel

16. In amphistomosis, which of the following stages are highly pathogenic

A. Adult flukes B. Immature flukes

C. Cercaria D. Eggs

17. The only amphistome present in liver and bile duct of ruminants is

A. *Gastrothylax crumenifer*

B. *Cotylophoron cotylophoron*

C. *Gigantocotyle explanatum*

D. *Paramphistomum cervi*

18. "Plug Feeding" is characteristic of

A. Immature Liver flukes B. Immature Amphistomes

C. Adult Liver flukes D. Adult Schistosomes

19. The sporangia of the fungus "*Pilobolus*" is involved in the transmission of

A. Ascarid worms B. Eye worms

C. Lung worms D. Stomach worms

20. Hydatidosis occurs by

A. Accidental ingestion of eggs of *Echinococcus granulosus*

B. Ingestion of fertile hydatid cyst fluid with ulcers in the intestine

C. Spillage of fertile hydatid cyst fluid on cut wounds in hands and fingers during slaughter of infected animals

D. All the above

21. Mclean county system is a sanitation method where pregnant animals are scrubbed to get rid of eggs and washed thoroughly. This is used for the control of

    A. *Parascaris equorum* B. *Toxocara vitulorum*
    C. *Ascaris suum* D. *Toxocara canis*

22. Red Maasai sheep of Kenya are resistant to

    A. Amphistomes
    B. Liver flukes
    C. Gastrointestinal nematodes especially *Haemonchus contortus*
    D. Ticks

23. Intermediate host for *Habronema majus* is

    A. Mosquito
    B. House fly
    C. Stable fly
    D. Black fly

24. The nematode without spicules is

    A. *Haemonchus contortus* B. *Mecistocirrus digitatus*
    C. *Trichinella spiralis* D. *Dictyocaulus viviparus*

25. Which of the following animal is not definitive host for *Protostrongylus rufescens*

    A. Sheep B. Goat
    C. Deer D. Cattle

26. Arecanut is used in the treatment of

    A. Trematodes B. Cestodes
    C. Nematodes D. All the above

27. Pick out the odd tapeworm
    A. *Dipylidium caninum*
    B. *Davainea proglottina*
    C. *Cotugnia digonopora*
    D. *Raillietina echinobothridia*

28. Nematodes
    A. Have both direct and indirect life cycle
    B. Are unsegmented and cylindrical
    C. Have sexual dimorphism
    D. All the above

29. Largest ascarid among the following is
    A. *Toxocara vitulorum*
    B. *Ascaris suum*
    C. *Parascaris equorum*
    D. *Ascaridia galli*

30. Important helminth responsible for calfhood mortality especially in buffalo calves is
    A. *Toxocara vitulorum*
    B. *Fasciola gigantica*
    C. *Haemonchus placei*
    D. *Strongyloides papillosus*

31. Which of the following is an *in vivo* test for detection of anthelmintic resistance?
    A. Egg hatch assay
    B. Tubulin binding assay
    C. Faecal egg count reduction test
    D. Larval paralysis assay

32. Tubulin binding assay is used to detect resistance against
    A. Ivermectin
    B. Levamisole
    C. Benzimidazoles
    D. Morantel

33. Which of the following practices lead to development of anthelmintic resistance?

    A. Underdosing

    B. Use of same anthelmintic frequently

    C. Faulty drenching equipments

    D. All the above

34. Which of the following practice will help to prevent the development of anthelmintic resistance?

    A. Overdosing

    B. Rotating anthelmintic groups

    C. Deworming all animals irrespective of worm load

    D. Continuous use of the same anthelmintic

❑❑❑

Chapter 23

# Frequently Asked Subjective Questions

## Short Notes

1. Cercarial dermatitis/Swimmer's itch/Clam digger's itch/Rice-paddy itch/Lakeside disease
2. Gid/Sturdy/Staggers
3. Nasal granuloma
4. Parasitic immunity
5. SNOAPAD
6. Pimply gut/Knotty gut
7. Visceral larval migrans
8. Anthelmintics and their mode of action
9. Mode of transmission of parasitic infections
10. Hepatitis cysticercosa
11. Poultry tapeworms
12. Gape worm of poultry
13. Self cure phenomenon
14. Periparturient rise
15. Crisis

16. Cutaneous larval migrans
17. Bladderworm stages of tapeworms
18. Hydatidosis
19. Kumri/Cerebrospinal nematodiasis
20. Clay pipe cirrhosis
21. Echinococcosis
22. Snoring disease
23. Snail control methods
24. Equine tapeworms
25. Gillor/Pitto/Immature amphistomosis
26. Broad fish tapeworm
27. Ascarids of dogs and cats
28. Milk spot liver
29. McLean County system
30. Thumps
31. Ascarid infection in equines
32. Ascarid infection in pigs
33. Poultry ascarids
34. Pin worm of horses
35. Life cycle of *Strongyloides papillosus*
36. *Chabertia ovina*
37. Hookworms of ruminants
38. Summer sore
39. Thorny headed worms
40. Life cycle patterns of helminths
41. Worm nest
42. Endectocides
43. Rules governing naming of parasites

44. Methods of application of antiparasitic drugs
45. Summer bleeding
46. Ear sore in buffaloes
47. Husk/Hoose/Parasitic bronchitis
48. DICTOL and DIFIL
49. Actinobody
50. ICZN

## Essay

1. Describe in detail the pathogenesis, clinical signs, treatment and control of haemonchosis in sheep
2. List out the amphistomes affecting ruminants. Write an essay on the pathogenesis, clinical signs, treatment and control of immature amphistomosis
3. List out the schistosomes affecting livestock. Describe in detail about life cycle, pathogenesis, treatment and control of Nasal schistosomosis in cattle
4. Write an essay on Harmful effects of parasites
5. Describe in detail about the life cycle, pathogenesis, treatment and control of Fasciolosis in sheep
6. List out the tapeworms of dogs. Describe in detail about life cycle, pathogenesis, zoonotic importance, clinical signs, treatment and control of *Echinococcus granulosus*
7. List out the gastrointestinal nematodes of ruminants. Write in detail about parasitic gastroenteritis
8. List out the tapeworms of ruminants. Write a detailed note on life cycle, pathogenesis, treatment and control of Monieziosis in sheep.
9. List out the tapeworms affecting poultry with their location and intermediate hosts. Describe the pathogenesis, treatment and control of poultry tapeworms
10. List out the ascarids affecting livestock. Write in detail about the life cycle, mode of transmission, pathogenesis, clinical signs, treatment and control of *Toxocara vitulorum* infection in calves

11. List out the strongyles affecting horses. Write a detailed note on morphology, life cycle, pathogenesis, clinical signs, treatment and control of *Strongylus vulgaris*
12. Ennumerate the hookworms affecting domestic animals. Write in detail about Ancylostomosis in dogs
13. List out the ascarids affecting dogs and cats. Write in detail about the life cycle, mode of transmission, pathogenesis, clinical signs, treatment and control of Toxocariasis in dogs with a note on its zoonotic importance
14. List out the filarid nematodes affecting animals. Write in detail about the life cycle, pathogenesis, clinical signs, treatment and control of the heartworm of dogs
15. List out the spirurid nematodes affecting animals. Write in detail about the life cycle, pathogenesis, clinical signs, treatment and control of *Spirocerca lupi*
16. Write an essay on various types of Immunity to parasitic infections
17. Describe in detail about Stomach worms of horses
18. List out the anthelmintics used in the treatment of trematode, cestode and nematode infections with their dose and route of administration with a note on contraindications if any
19. List the tapeworms of zoonotic importance. Describe their bladder worm stages and give an account of *Echinococcus granulosus*
20. List out the lung worms affecting ruminants. Write in detail about the life cycle, pathogenesis, clinical signs, treatment, vaccination and control of lung worm infections in ruminants
21. Give an account of PGE

Chapter 24

# Important Text Books in General Veterinary Parasitology & Helminthology

1. Helminths, Arthropods and Protozoa of domesticated animals: EJL Soulsby
2. Veterinary Parasitology: G.M. Urquhart, J. Armour, J.L. Duncan, A.M. Dunn, F.W. Jenning
3. Georgi's Parasitology for Veterinarians: Dwight D. Bowman
4. Veterinary Helminthology: Tibor Kassai
5. Veterinary Parasitology: M.A. Taylor, R.L. Koop, R.L. Wall
6. Parasitic infections of domestic animals: A Diagnostic Manual: Johannes Kaufmann
7. Veterinary Helminthology: S.C. Mandal

□□□

Chapter 25

# Answers
# Fill Up the Blanks

## General Veterinary Parasitology

1. Autoheteroxenous
2. Carl Linnaeus
3. Stenoxenous
4. Aestivation
5. Monoxenous or Homoxenous
6. Vector
7. Phoresy
8. Homospecific or Homogenetic
9. Carrier
10. Specific
11. Zooanthroponoses
12. Sporadic
13. Symbiosis
14. Predatorism/Predation
15. Cyclical or Biological
16. Convalescent carrier host

17. Commensalism
18. Paratenic host
19. Zoonoses
20. Mechanical
21. Euryxenous
22. Sterile or Complete or Sterilizing
23. Parasitiasis, Parasitosis
24. Contact carrier
25. Underlined, Italizised
26. Taxonomy
27. Symbiosis
28. Trans stadial
29. Anthropozoonoses
30. Saprozoic
31. Diapause
32. Commensalism
33. Concomitant immunity
34. Systematics
35. Veterinary Parasitology
36. Intermittent or Periodic or Occasional
37. Parasitism
38. Premunity or infection immunity or incomplete immunity or non sterilizing immunity
39. Hibernation or Winter sleep
40. Stenoxenous
41. Prenatal or transplacental
42. Rhode island red, Plymouth Rock
43. Transport

44. Active, Passive
45. Congenital
46. Natural, Artificial
47. Incidental
48. Transcolostral or Transmammary
49. Parasitos, para-besides, sitos-food
50. Temporary
51. Law of Priority
52. Holozoic
53. More
54. Hyperparasite
55. Heterogenetic or Heterospecific
56. Uninomial, Binomial, Trinomial nomenclature
57. Relative
58. Schizogony
59. Hypobiosis
60. Sporogony
61. Incubation period
62. Definitive host
63. Transovarian transmission
64. Capital, Small
65. Parasite
66. Ectoparasite, Endoparasite
67. Immunity
68. Gametogony
69. Host, Locality
70. Indirect
71. Nomenclature

72. Protelean parasite
73. Pandemic
74. Acquired or Induced
75. Reservoir host
76. Host
77. Ida, oidea, inae
78. Obligatory
79. Parasitology
80. Facultative heteroxenous, Obligatory heteroxenous
81. Pseudoparasite/ Artifact
82. Infection, Infestation
83. Paedogenesis
84. Heterogenetic
85. Epidemic or Epizootic
86. Ecology
87. Prepatent period or Biological incubation period
88. Threshold value
89. Dung or faeces or dropping
90. Intercalary host
91. Commensalism
92. Standardized nomenclature for animal parasitic diseases
93. IgE
94. Eosinophils
95. Symbiosis or Symbiotic relationship
96. Symbiont
97. Parasite, Host
98. Hyperinfection
99. Bearer

100. Epidemiology
101. 10, 40
102. Isohaemagglutinins
103. Opsonins
104. Ablastins
105. Concealed/hidden

## Helminthology

### *Trematodes*

1. *Dicrocoelium dendriticum*, cercaria
2. Immature amphistomes
3. *Fasciolopsis buski*
4. Niclosamide (60 mg/kg po), Praziquantel (20 mg/kg po)
5. *Opisthorchis tenuicollis*
6. Worm
7. Schistosomes
8. Parenchyma
9. Holes
10. Oral sucker, acetabulum
11. Identification
12. Shell gland
13. Light, temperature, salinity of water
14. Miracidium, sporocyst, redia, cercaria, metacercaria
15. Sporocyst
16. Snail
17. Redia, metacercaria
18. Xiphidocercous
19. Composite, hexagonal
20. Acute, chronic

21. Acute fasciolosis
22. Stage of cellular infiltration, stage of actinobody formation, stage of abscess formation
23. Amphistomes
24. *Gigantocotyle explanatum*
25. Fasciolosis
26. Snails
27. *Opisthorchis tenuicollis*
28. *Paragonimus westermanii*
29. Gynaecophoric canal
30. Miracidium, Cercaria
31. Fasciolosis
32. Solenocytes
33. 3 hours
34. 1-6, polyembryony
35. Daughter redia
36. Cystogenous
37. Pearly/milky white
38. Snails
39. *Fasciolopsis buski*
40. *Paragonimus westermanii*
41. Right caudal
42. Immature amphistomosis
43. Immature amphistomes
44. Oxyclozanide, Tetramisole
45. Blood
46. Blood vessels
47. *Schistosoma spindale*
48. *Schistosoma spindale*
49. *Schistosoma spindale*

## Cestodes

1. *Moniezia* sp.
2. *Diphyllobothrium latum*
3. *Diphyllobothrium latum*
4. *Taenia solium*/Pork tapeworm of man
5. Fertile, sterile
6. *Taenia solium*
7. Poultry
8. *Stilesia hepatica*
9. *Echinococcus granulosus*
10. *Davainea proglottina*
11. *Taenia sp., Dipylidium caninum*
12. Hydatidosis/Cystic echinococcosis
13. Coracidium, Procercoid, Pleurocercoid
14. Tapeworms
15. Hydatidosis
16. Tape like structure
17. Saprozoic
18. Head/Scolex, Neck and Body/Strobila
19. Suckers, bothria
20. Suckers, bothria
21. Rostellum
22. Armed, unarmed
23. Proglottids
24. Single, double
25. Lateral, ventral
26. Immature, mature and gravid
27. Cotyloda

28. Gravid
29. Apolysis
30. Anapolysis
31. Onchosphere, hexacanth (6 hooked) embryo
32. Outer capsule, outer envelope, inner envelope, onchosphere membrane
33. Coracidium
34. Metacestode/bladder worm stage
35. Cysticercus
36. Cysticercoid
37. Strobilocercous
38. Coenurus
39. Hydatid cyst
40. Hydatid sand
41. Procercoid, pleurocercoid
42. Procercoid, pleurocercoid
43. Tetrathyridium
44. 1, 2
45. Triangular, square
46. Pyriform
47. *Raillietina echinobothridia*
48. *Amoebotaenia sphenoides*
49. *Davainea proglottina*
50. *Dipylidium caninum*
51. *Dipylidium caninum*
52. Taenid
53. *Cysticercus tenuicollis*
54. Brain and spinal cord, subcutaneous tissue

55. *Coenurus cerebralis*
56. *Echinococcus granulosus*
57. *Echinococcus granulosus*
58. Inner germinal
59. Anaphylactic shock
60. *Echinococcus granulosus*
61. Hydatid cyst
62. 2.5-10% formalin
63. Albendazole, Mebendazole
64. 4-8
65. Heart, masseter muscle
66. Brain, subcutaneous tissue, eye
67. *Diphyllobothrium latum*

## Nematodes

1. *Strongyloides papillosus*
2. *Spirocerca lupi*
3. *Oesophagostomum columbianum, Oesophagostomum radiatum*
4. *Toxocara canis*
5. *Spirocerca lupi*
6. *Haemonchus contortus*
7. Visceral larval migrans/Ocular larval migrans, *Toxocara canis*
8. *Ancylostoma caninum*
9. Gastrointestinal nematodes
10. *Toxocara canis, Ancylostoma caninum*
11. Geographical information systems
12. Quantitative, EPG (egg per gram of faeces), OPG (oocyst per gram of faeces)
13. Microfilaria

14. Ivermectin
15. Microfilaria
16. *Haemonchus contortus*
17. 36
18. *Heterakis gallinarum*
19. *Dracunculus medinensis*
20. Teratogenicity
21. *Haemonchus contortus*
22. Baermann
23. Strongyle
24. Strongyle
25. *Ascaridia galli*
26. FAMACHA
27. Trichinoscope
28. Cuticle
29. *Tetrameres sp, Oesophagostomum sp.*
30. Alae
31. Cervical alae, Caudal alae
32. Pseudocoelom
33. *Gongylonema sp.*
34. *Physaloptera sp*
35. Hypodermis
36. Ascarid
37. Leaf crown
38. External leaf crown, Internal leaf crown
39. Hook worms
40. *Heterakis gallinarum*
41. Rhabditiform, Filariform

42. Rhabditiform
43. Filariform
44. Osmoregulation
45. Amphids and Phasmids
46. Smaller
47. Spicules
48. Gubernaculum, telamon
49. *Haemonchus contortus*
50. Oviparous, ovoviviparous, viviparous
51. Oviparous
52. Ovoviviparous
53. Viviparous
54. Filarid
55. *Oxyuris equi, Trichuris sp*
56. Morula, tadpole
57. Ascarids
58. *Spirocerca lupi*
59. Strongyle
60. Temperature, moisture, larval movement and enzymes secreted by larva
61. CO2 concentration
62. Moulting or ecdysis
63. 4
64. Egg containing L2
65. Strongylidae and Trichostrongylidae
66. *Ancylostoma and Bunostomum sp*
67. Metastrongylidae and *Habronema*
68. *Setaria digitata* or *Dirofilaria immitis*

69. 2 lakhs
70. Ascarids
71. $8^{th}$
72. *Toxocara vitulorum*
73. Direct, Prenatal, Transmammary, Paratenic host
74. Pups up to 3 months age, somatic migration
75. $42^{nd}$ day
76. Transmammary
77. Rodents
78. Direct and paratenic host
79. *Toxocara canis*
80. Earthworm
81. Young (1-3 months old)
82. *Ascaridia galli*
83. Goblet
84. *Ascaridia galli*
85. *Ascaridia galli*
86. *Heterakis gallinarum*
87. *Oxyuris equi*
88. Pin
89. *Strongyloides*
90. *Strongyloides*
91. Heterogonic, homogonic
92. *Strongyloides stercoralis, Strongyloides avium*
93. Bursate nematodes
94. Dorsal gutter
95. Strongyles
96. Corona radiata

97. Bursal rays
98. Negatively, positively
99. Dawn, dusk
100. *Oesophagostomum columbianum/Haemonchus contortus*
101. *Chabertia ovina*
102. *Chabertia ovina*
103. Earthworm, snail and slug
104. *Stephanurus dentatus*
105. Hook
106. 8 cell
107. 16,000
108. Oral ingestion, skin penetration
109. Oral ingestion, skin penetration, prenatal and transmammary
110. *Ancylostoma caninum*
111. 0.001 ml
112. Microcytic hypochromic
113. Common salt, sodium borate
114. *Agriostomum vryburgi*
115. *Trichostrongylus sp.*
116. 0.05 ml
117. Hyperacute
118. Acute
119. Chronic
120. *Haemonchus contortus*
121. L3 Larvae
122. *Nematodirus spathiger*
123. Periparturient rise
124. Biohelminths, Geohelminths

125. *Dictyocaulus sp.*
126. *Dictyocaulus viviparus, Dictyocaulus filaria*
127. *Mullerius capillaris*
128. Earthworm
129. *Metastrogylus elongatus*
130. *Draschia megastoma*
131. *Draschia megastoma*
132. Goats
133. *Spirocerca lupi*
134. Disophenol, Diethylcarbamazine, Ivermectin, Albendazole
135. *Tetrameres mohtedai*
136. *Physaloptera praeputialis*
137. *Gnathosoma spinigerum*
138. *Gnathosoma spinigerum*
139. Sausage
140. 2% formalin, methylene blue
141. Diethylcarbamazine (DEC)
142. *Dirofilaria repens, Dipetalonema reconditum*
143. *Setaria digitata*
144. *Dracunculus medinensis*
145. *Dioctophyma renale*
146. Saprophytic
147. Acanthor, Uterine bell
148. Cystacanth
149. Fumarate reductase system and Tubulin binding
150. Nerve ganglion stimulation and depolarizing neuromuscular system
151. Acetylcholinesterase

152. Uncoupling mitochondrial reaction
153. Avermectins (Ivermectin, Doramectin etc.)
154. Office International Des Epizooties
155. Food and Agricultural Organization
156. World Health Organization
157. International Laboratory for Research on Animal Diseases, Nairobi

     (Kenya)
158. Biotechnology and Biological Research Council, London, United Kingdom
159. Indian Council of Agricultural Research, New Delhi
160. Anthelmintic resistance
161. Faecal egg count reduction test (FECRT), Controlled test
162. Targeted selective treatment
163. FAMACHA chart

# ANSWERS
# MULTIPLE CHOICE QUESTIONS

## General Veterinary Parasitology

| | |
|---|---|
| 1. C | 2. D |
| 3. D | 4. D |
| 5. B | 6. D |
| 7. D | 8. B |
| 9. D | 10. C |
| 11. D | 12. C |
| 13. D | 14. C |
| 15. B | 16. C |
| 17. D | 18. C |

| | |
|---|---|
| 19. D | 20. B |
| 21. A | 22. C |
| 23. B | 24. A |
| 25. B | 26. B |
| 27. D | 28. C |
| 29. A | 30. D |
| 31. B | 32. B |

## Helminthology

| | |
|---|---|
| 1. D | 2. C |
| 3. C | 4. B |
| 5. C | 6. D |
| 7. B | 8. C |
| 9. B | 10. C |
| 11. B | 12. C |
| 13. B | 14. C |
| 15. A | 16. B |
| 17. C | 18. B |
| 19. C | 20. D |
| 21. C | 22. C |
| 23. C | 24. C |
| 25. D | 26. B |
| 27. A | 28. D |
| 29. C | 30. A |
| 31. C | 32. C |
| 33. D | 34. B |

PART-II

# VETERINARY ENTOMOLOGY AND ACAROLOGY

Chapter 1

# Common Name and Scientific Name of Insects and Acarines

| S.No. | Common name | Scientific name |
|---|---|---|
| 1. | Dappled mosquito | *Anopheles* |
| 2. | Tiger mosquito | *Aedes* |
| 3. | Biting midges/Punkies/ No see ums | *Culicoides* spp. |
| 4. | Black fly/Buffalo gnat/ Turkey gnat/ Potu fly | *Simulium* spp. |
| 5. | Sand fly/Owl midges | *Phlebotomus* spp. |
| 6. | Horse fly/Breeze fly/ Green head fly/Gad fly/ March fly/Blind fly | *Tabanus striatus* |
| 7. | Horse stomach bot fly/ Intestinal bot fly | *Gasterophilus* spp. |
| 8. | Grubs | *Larvae of Gasterophilus, Oestrus ovis, Hypoderma lineatum* |
| 9. | Sheep Nasal fly/Sheep head fly/ Sheep nasal bot fly | *Oestrus ovis* |
| 10. | Ox warble fly/Heel fly/ Common cattle grub fly | *Hypoderma bovis, Hypoderma lineatum* |
| 11. | House fly/Picnic fly/ Enteric fly | *Musca domestica* |

| | | |
|---|---|---|
| 12. | Stable fly/Dog fly/Biting house fly/Barn fly | *Stomoxys calcitrans* |
| 13. | Blow fly/Bottle fly | *Calliphora* spp., *Lucilia* spp., *Chrysomia* spp. |
| 14. | Blue Bottle fly | *Calliphora* spp. |
| 15. | Green Bottle fly/ Copper bottle fly | *Lucilia* spp. |
| 16. | Blue Green bottle fly/ Old world screw worm fly | *Chrysomia bezziana* |
| 17. | Flesh fly | *Sarcophaga* spp. |
| 18. | Sheep ked/Sheep tick fly | *Melophagus ovinus* |
| 19. | Forest fly/Louse fly | *Hipposboscidae* *Hippobosca maculata* |
| 20. | Pigeon fly | *Pseudolynchia maura* *(Pseudolynchia canariensis)* |
| 21. | Bed bug | *Cimex* spp. |
| 22. | Kissing bug/Cone nosed bug/Assassin bug/ Reduvid bug | *Triatoma sp.* |
| 23. | Short nosed cattle louse | *Haematopinus eurysternus* |
| 24. | Long nosed cattle louse/ Blue louse of cattle | *Linognathus vituli* |
| 25. | Wing louse of poultry | *Lipeurus caponis* |
| 26. | Shaft louse of poultry | *Menopon gallinae* |
| 27. | Yellow Body louse of poultry/Chicken body louse | *Menacanthus stramineus* |
| 28. | Chewing louse of dog | *Trichodectes canis* *Heterodoxus spiniger* |
| 29. | Dog flea | *Ctenocephalides canis* |
| 30. | Cat flea | *Ctenocephalides felis* |
| 31. | Tail switch louse of cattle | *Haematopinus quadripertusus* |
| 32. | Hog louse/Pig louse/ Largest livestock louse | *Haematopinus suis* |
| 33. | Cattle louse | *Haematopinus eurysternus* |

| | | |
|---|---|---|
| 34. | Buffalo louse | *Haematopinus tuberculatus* |
| 35. | Foot louse of sheep | *Linognathus pedalis* |
| 36. | Goat sucking louse | *Linognathus stenopsis* |
| 37. | Human head louse | *Pediculus humanus capitus* |
| 38. | Human pubic louse/ Crab louse | *Phthirus pubis* |
| 39. | Stick tight flea/Stick fast flea/Fowl flea/ Chicken flea | *Echidnophaga gallinacea* |
| 40. | Oriental rat flea/Black flea | *Xenopsylla cheopis* |
| 41. | Human flea | *Pulex irritans* |
| 42. | Fowl tick/Blue tick/ Abode tick/Blue bug/ Chicken tick | *Argas persicus* |
| 43. | Spinose ear tick | *Otobius megnini* |
| 44. | Eyed Tampan/Sand tampan/Sand tick | *Ornithodoros savignyi* |
| 45. | Castor bean tick | *Ixodes ricinus* |
| 46. | Cattle tick | *Rhipicephalus* (*Boophilus*) *annulatus*, *Rhipicephalus* (*Boophilus*) *microplus* |
| 47. | Bont leg tick | *Hyalomma marginatum* |
| 48. | Brown dog tick/Kennel tick | *Rhipicephalus sanguineus* |
| 49. | Bont tick | *Amblyomma hebraeum* |
| 50. | Lone star tick | *Amblyomma americanum* |
| 51. | Ear mite of dog | *Otodectes cynotis* |
| 52. | Red mite of poultry/ Roost mite of poultry/ Chicken mite | *Dermanyssus gallinae* |
| 53. | Tropical fowl mite | *Ornithonyssus bursa* |
| 54. | Feather mite of poultry | *Megninia ginglymura* |
| 55. | Goat follicular mite | *Demodex caprae* |
| 56. | Tongue worm | *Linguatula serrata* |
| 57. | New world screw worm fly | *Cochliomyia hominivorax* |

| | | |
|---|---|---|
| 58. | Dog sucking louse | *Linognathus setosus* |
| 59. | Goat biting louse | *Damalinia caprae* |
| 60. | Cattle biting louse/ Red louse | *Damalinia bovis (Bovicola bovis)* |
| 61. | Human body louse | *Pediculus humanus corporis* |
| 62. | Eyeless tampan | *Ornithodoros moubata* |
| 63. | Chewing louse of cat | *Felicola subrostratus* |
| 64. | Sheep scab mite | *Psoroptes ovis* |
| 65. | Follicular mite of dog | *Demodex canis* |
| 66. | Velvet mite/Trombiculid mite | *Trombicula autumnalis* |
| 67. | Chicken head louse | *Cuclotogaster heterographus* |
| 68. | Large chicken louse | *Goniocotes gigas* |
| 69. | Fluff louse of poultry | *Goniocotes gallinae* |
| 70. | Buffalo fly/Horn fly | *Haematobia exigua* |
| 71. | Biting louse of sheep/ Little red louse of sheep | *Damalinia ovis* |

□□□

Chapter 2

# Habitat/Breeding Sites of Insects

| S.No. | Insect | Habitat/Breeding site(s) |
|---|---|---|
| 1. | *Anopheles* mosquito | Fresh water such as irrigation water, rain water, ponds, rivers etc. |
| 2. | *Aedes* mosquito | Stored water such as in buckets, tree holes, discarded tyres etc. |
| 3. | *Culex* mosquito | Contaminated water with high organic content such as water in drains, ditches etc. |
| 4. | *Phelebotomus* sp. | Cracks, crevices, holes in walls, rocks, Non aquatic areas where it is dark, moist with decaying organic material |
| 5. | *Culicoides* sp. | Moist decaying material, ecotone between terrestrial and aquatic habitat |
| 6. | *Simulium* sp. | Fluvial ecosystem-swiftly running water, splash zone |
| 7. | *Tabanus* | Hemihydrobiont- soil near the water |
| 8. | *Musca domestica* | Garbage, manure-horse dung preferred, decaying organic debris, Poultry manure, human excreta, abundant in rainy season |
| 9. | *Stomoxys calcitrans* | Bedding material of horses contaminated with urine |

| | | |
|---|---|---|
| 10. | *Haematobia exigua* | Dung |
| 11. | *Chrysomyia bezziana* | Wounds on animals |
| 12. | *Chrysomyia megacephala* | Carcass |
| 13. | *Lucilia* sp. | Live animals on wounds, organic debris |
| 14. | *Sarcophaga dux* | Flesh |
| 15. | *Oestrus ovis* | Deposit larvae on the muzzle of sheep |
| 16. | *Hypoderma lineatum* | Lays eggs on the hairs in the heel of cattle |
| 17. | *Gasterophilus equi* | Eggs on the hairs on fetlock of horses |
| 18. | *Hippobosca sp.* | Dung |
| 19. | *Melophagus ovinus* | On the host |
| 20. | *Ctenocephalides felis* | Eggs on the ground |
| 21. | Ticks | Off the host, in the habitat off the host |
| 22. | Mites | On the host |
| 23. | Bugs | Off the host in cracks and crevices |

□□□

Chapter 3

# Important Morphological Characters of Eggs of Insects

| S.No. | Insect | Characters of egg |
|---|---|---|
| 1. | *Anopheles* sp. | Boat-shaped egg having a pair of frilled lateral expansions called 'floats'.<br>Eggs laid singly |
| 2. | *Culex* sp. | Large number of spindle shaped eggs clumped together in the form of an "egg raft" with the pointed end towards the surface of water |
| 3. | *Aedes* sp. | Spindle shaped reticulated egg without floats (laid singly) |
| 4. | *Phlebotomus* sp. | Yellowish in colour when laid which turns dark brown<br>Show the presence of shining longitudinal black wavy lines, raised slightly and joined by slender cross lines<br>40-50 eggs are laid in a lifetime by the female fly |
| 5. | *Culicoides* sp. | Eggs 0.5 mm long<br>Small, cigar or banana shaped, cylindrical, curved and dark in colour |
| 6. | *Simulium* sp. | Long ovoid triangular in shape<br>Smooth surface, pale often whitish but darkens to brown or black colour.<br>Covered with gelatinous material |

| | | |
|---|---|---|
| 7. | *Tabanus* | Laid in masses of 200-1000, glued to the surface of substrate especially vegetation overhanging water |
| | | Creamy white in colour, become darker later on |
| | | Stratified into 2-3 layers |
| | | Cigar shaped and water proofed |
| 8. | *Musca domestica* | 100-150 eggs are laid at a time and an average of 600/lifetime |
| | | Elongate creamy white, oval/banana shaped/ 1 mm long with two ridge like thickenings on the dorsal aspect- the hatching pleat |
| | | Singly laid |
| 9. | *Stomoxys calcitrans* | 25- 50 eggs are laid after blood meal |
| | | Eggs are dirty white or yellow in colour, 1 mm, with only one dorsal ridge or hatching pleat |
| 10. | *Haematobia exigua* | Similar to *Stomoxys* sp. |
| 11. | *Hypoderma lineatum* | Spindle shaped |
| | | Provided with a clasper with the help of which they hold on to the hair |
| 12. | *Ctenocephalides felis* | Large pearly white, glistening and oval in shape |
| | | 200 eggs produced in 2-4 days time |
| | | Eggs may be sticky or dry |
| 13. | *Cimex sp.* | Eggs are creamy white |
| | | 1 mm long with an operculum |
| 14. | Lice eggs (Nits) | Eggs are operculated without stalk |
| | | Cemented to hairs or feathers |
| 15. | Tick eggs | Eggs are laid in thousands in masses |
| | | Small reddish brown in colour and glistening covered by waxy layer |

❑❑❑

Chapter 4

# Identification of Insects Based on Wing Venation/ Characteristics

| S.No. | Wing venation/Characteristics | Insect |
|---|---|---|
| 1. | Wings are narrow, lanceolate and bears scales<br>Wing venation is characteristic in that the 2nd, 4th and 5th longitudinal veins are forked | Mosquitoes-culicines |
| 2. | Accumulation of scales at the anterior border of the wing giving it a dappled appearance | Anopheline mosquitoes |
| 3. | Wings large lanceolate, held roof like over the abodomen. 2nd longitudinal vein forked twice | *Phlebotomus* fly |
| 4. | Wings folded over the abdomen, with light and dark pattern, due to pigmentation in the wing membrane-grey with pale spots covered with minute setae (blotched wing) | *Culicoides* sp. |
| 5. | Forking of the third longitudinal vein | *Tabanus* sp. |
| 6. | Wing venation is characteristic in that the 4th longitudinal vein curves upwards at about the middle and joins the 3rd vein to form the closed apical cell | *Musca domestica* |

| | | |
|---|---|---|
| 7. | The apical cell is open<br>Wing kept at divergent angle | *Stomoxys calcitrans* |
| 8. | Wing shows the presence of a dark, irregular transverse band running across it | *Gasterophilus equi* |
| 9. | Wings when present have a characteristic venation- veins crowded in the anterior margin while the posterior portion reveals fine wrinkling | *Hippobosca and Pseudolynchia* |

□□□

Chapter 5

# Identification of Insects Based on Arista

**S.No.** **Arista** **Insect/Brief description**

1.

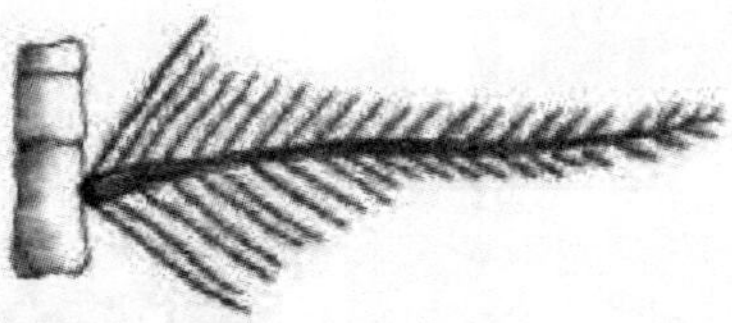

*Musca domestica*

- Bilaterally plumed upto the tip

2.

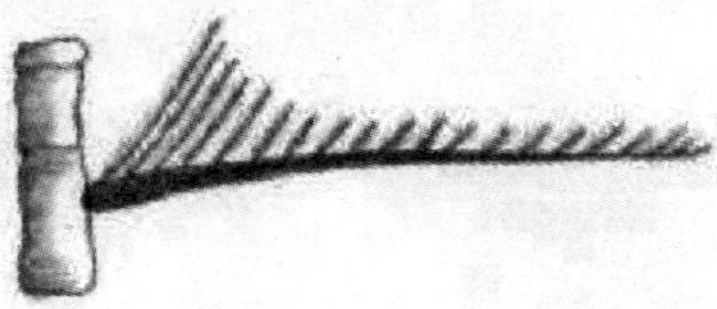

*Stomoxys calcitrans*

- Presence of bristles only on the dorsal aspect
- Having 8-10 bristles

3.

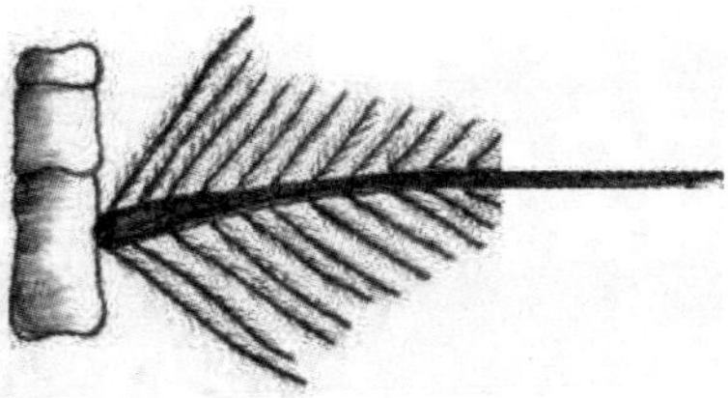

*Sarcophaga* sp.

- Arista bilaterally plumose upto the middle and bare beyond

4.

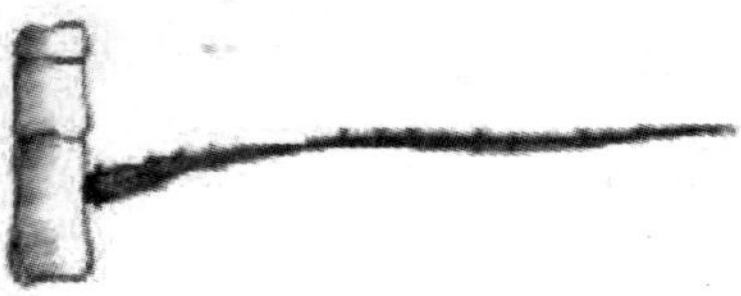

*Oestrus ovis*

- Bare arista

❑❑❑

Chapter 6

# Identification of Insect Larvae Based on Posterior Spiracles

| S.No. | Posterior spiracle | Insect Larva |
|---|---|---|
| 1. | 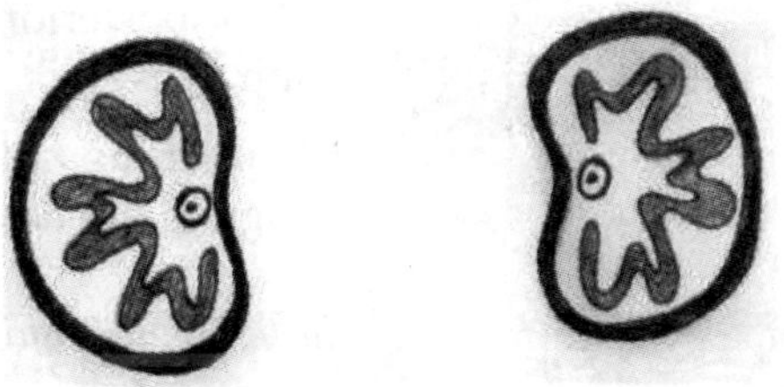 | *Musca* sp.<br>• A pair of brown 'D' shaped spiracles<br>• A chitnised ring (button) and 3 sinuous 'm' shaped stigmatic slits in each spiracle |
| 2. | 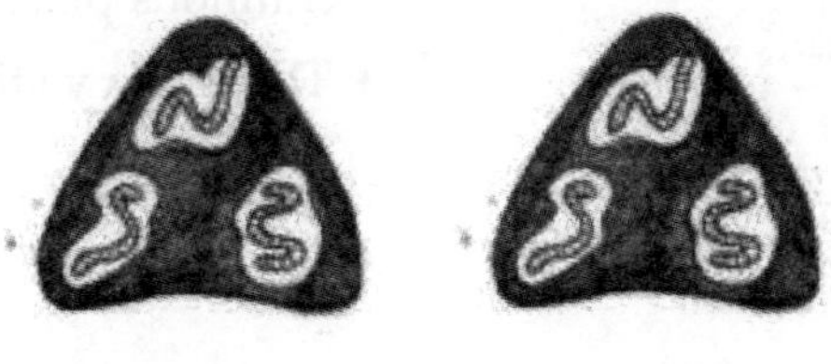 | *Stomoxys calcitrans*<br>• Roughly triangular in shape<br>• Three 'S' shaped slits in each stigmal plate of the spiracles |
| 3. | 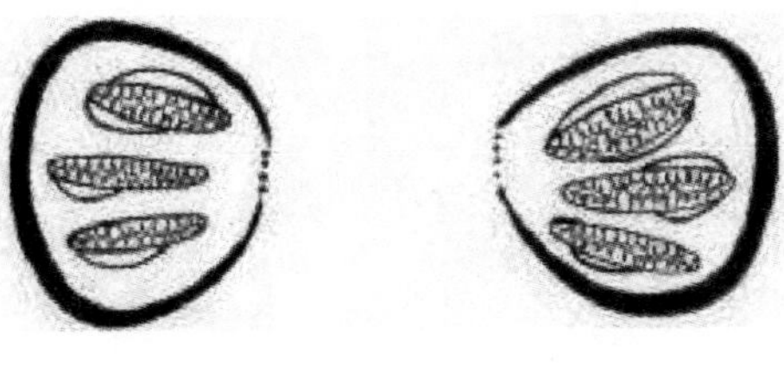 | *Chrysomyia* sp.<br>• A pair of more or less circular spiracles with three longitudinal slits<br>• Incomplete peritreme |

4.

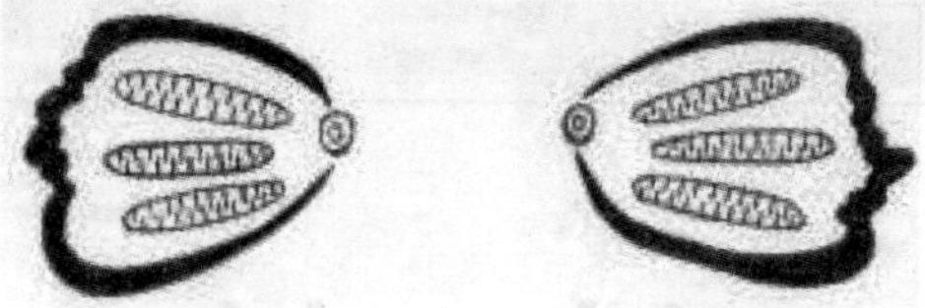

*Sarcophaga sp.*

- Incomplete circumference
- Presence of button
- Three longitudinal slits

5.

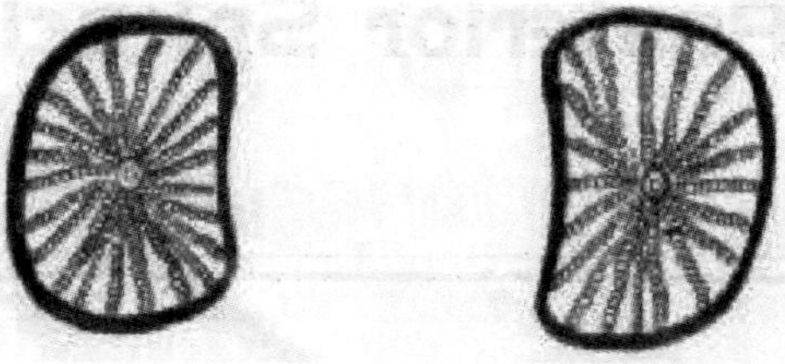

*Oestrus ovis*

- Large somewhat 'D' shaped dark chitinous plates
- A central and numerous accessory spiracular openings

6.

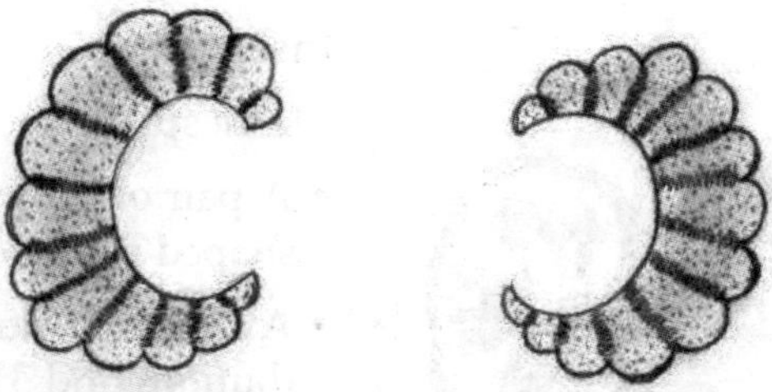

*Hypoderma lineatum*

- Kidney shaped very dark posterior spiracles
- Numerous radiating stigmal openings

7.

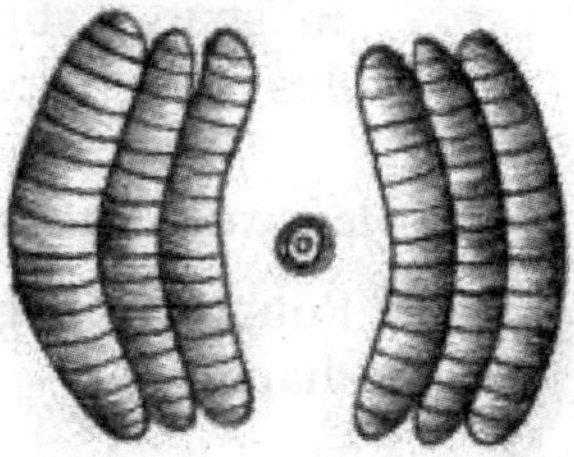

*Gasterophilus equi*

- Bean-shaped brownish chitinous plates
- Three wavy stigmal slits

□□□

Chapter 7

# Vector Potentiality/ Pathological Conditions Caused by Insects

| S.No. | Insect | Diseases/Parasites transmitted/ Pathological conditions |
|---|---|---|
| 1. | *Anopheles stephensi* | Human malaria<br>*Setaria digitata*<br>*Dirofilaria immitis* |
| 2. | *Culicines- Culex and Aedes sp.* | ***Culex* spp.**<br>Japanese B encephalitis virus in children<br>***Aedes* spp.**<br>Yellow fever virus<br>Dengue hemorrhagic fever<br>Rift valley fever virus<br>Chikungunya fever virus<br>Both the genus are involved in transmission of *Dirofilaria immitis* in dogs, *Setaria digitata* in cattle, Eastern equine encephalitis virus and St. Louis encephalitis virus |
| 3. | *Phlebotomus argentipes*<br>*Phlebotomus sergenti* | *Leishmania donovani*<br>*Leishmania tropica* |
| 4. | *Simulium sp.* | Transmits *Leucocytozoon smithi* in turkeys and *L. simondi* in ducks |

| | | |
|---|---|---|
| | | Intermediate host for *Onchocerca gutturosa* in cattle and *O. volvulus* of man -the filarid is the cause of river blindness in man<br>It also transmits eastern equine encephalitis virus and vesicular stomatitis virus in cattle |
| 5. | *Culicoides sp.* | Blue tongue virus in sheep<br>African Horse sickness virus<br>Bovine ephemeral fever virus<br>Eastern equine encephalitis virus<br>*Leucocytozoon caulleryi* in fowls<br>*Haemoproteus nethionis* in ducks, geese etc.<br>They also act as intermediate host for filarid nematodes like *Onchocerca cervicalis* in horses and *O. gibsoni* in cattle<br>Cause allergic dermatitis in horses called sweet itch/ sweat itch/ Queensland itch/ Summer dermatitis |
| 6. | *Tabanus sp.* | Mechanical vector for *Trypanosoma evansi* and cyclical vector for *Trypanosoma theileri*<br>Mechanically they can also transmit *Anaplasma maginale* and the causative organisms of anthrax, tularaemia, rinderpest and equine infectious anaemia<br>Bites are painful and irritating and give rise to wheals<br>Animals become restless and unmanageable<br>Blood loss 0.35 ml/ day/ fly |
| 7. | *Musca domestica* | Bacterial diseases such as cholera, typhoid, paratyphoid, T.B., salmonella, *E.coli* dysentery, anthrax etc.,<br>Viral diseases such as poliomyelitis and infectious hepatitis<br>Protozoan diseases such as amoebic dysentery, giardiasis |

| | | |
|---|---|---|
| | | Acts as the intermediate host for *Habronema muscae, Draschia megastoma, Thelazia rhodesii, Raillietina spp., Choanotaenia infundibulum*<br>Mechanical transmission of the eggs of the following is also possible - *Taenia solium, Toxocara sp, Ancylostoma, Hymenolepis, Dipylidium caninum* and *Diphyllobothrium latum*<br>Causes nuisance, fly worry and causes specks on chicken eggs which reduces the shelf life of eggs |
| 8. | *Stomoxys calcitrans* | Mechanically transmits *Trypanosoma evansi*<br>Also is a mechanical vector for anthrax, rinderpest, tetanus bacteria and poliomyelitis virus<br>It is an intermediate host for *Habronema majus* |
| 9. | *Oestrus ovis* | False Gid/Sturdy/Snotty nose/Gadding in sheep |
| 10. | *Hypoderma lineatum* | Warbles/Butchers jelly/Licked beef in cattle |
| 11. | *Gasterophilus equi* | Intestinal myiasis in horses |
| 12. | *Chrysomyia, Lucilia* and *Sarcophaga* | Myiasis (*Lucilia cuprina* causes Strike in sheep) |
| 13. | *Hippobosca maculata* | Transmits *Trypanosoma theileri* cyclically to cattle |
| 14. | *Melophagus ovinus* | Transmits a non pathogenic *Trypanosoma melophagium*<br>Causes severe irritation leading to Cockle/Rib Cockle/Back loss in sheep |
| 15. | *Pseudolynchia canariensis (P.maura)* | *Hemoproteus columbae* |
| 16. | *Ctenocephalides felis felis, Ctenocephalides canis* | Intermediate host for the tapeworm of dogs - *Dipylidium caninum,* transmit a filarid worm of dogs - *Dipetalonema reconditum* |

| | | |
|---|---|---|
| 17. | *Ctenocephalides felis* | Causes flea hypersensitivity or flea bite dermatitis or Miliary dermatitis/Flea allergy |
| 18. | *Xenopsylla cheopis* | Transmits *Yersinia pestis* causing bubonic plague in human beings, endemic or murine exanthematous typhus caused by *Rickettsia mooseri* and tularaemia caused by *Francisella tularensis* |
| 19. | *Echidnophaga gallinacea* | Causes temporary blindness in chicken |
| 20. | *Argas persicus* | *Aegyptionella pullorum* and *Borrelia anserina* (Fowl Spirochaetosis)<br>Causes anemia and insomnia |
| 21. | *Otobius megnini* | Otacariasis<br>Ear canker |
| 22. | *Ornithodoros savignyi* | *Anaplasma marginale,* Spirochaetosis |
| 23. | *Rhipicephaus microplus* | *Babesia bigemina, Babesia bovis* |
| 24. | *Haemaphysalis bispinosa* | *Theileria mutans* |
| 25. | *Rhipicephalus sanguineus* | *Babesia canis, Babesia gibsoni, Hepatozoon canis and Ehrlichia canis* |
| 26. | *Dermacentor variabilis* | Rocky mountain spotted fever, Q fever, tularemia, causes tick paralysis |
| 27. | *Ixodes ricinus* | *Babesia divergens* |
| 28. | *Amblyomma maculatum* | Heart water disease in cattle caused by *Cowdria ruminantium* |
| 29. | *Hyalomma anatolicum, Hyalomma marginatum isaaci* | *Theileria annulata, T.orientalis, Anaplasma marginale, Ehrlichia bovis* |
| 30. | *Rhipicephalus haemaphysaloides* | *Babesia sp.* |
| 31. | *Sarcoptes scabiei* | Sarcoptic mange/Scabies in animals |
| 32. | *Psoroptes ovis* | Sheep scab |
| 33. | *Demodex canis* | Red Mange/Demodectic Mange/ Follicular Mange |
| 34. | *Psoroptes cuniculi* | Ear canker/Ear mange in rabbits |
| 35. | *Chorioptes equi* | Foot mange in horses |
| 36. | *Megninia ginglymura* | Depluming itch in poultry |

| | | |
|---|---|---|
| 37. | *Cnemidocoptes gallinae* | Depluming itch in poultry |
| 38. | *Cnemidocoptes mutans* | Scaly leg in poultry |
| 39. | Lice | Pediculosis/Lousiness |
| 40. | *Heterodoxus spiniger* | Act as intermediate host for *Dipylidium caninum* and *Dipetalonema reconditum* in dogs |
| 41. | *Haematopinus suis* | Transmits swine fever virus |
| 42. | *Cimex spp.* | Causes anemia and insomnia |
| 43. | *Cheyletiella parasitivorax* and *Cheyletiella yasguri* | Causes a condition called "Walking dandruff" |

❑❑❑

Chapter 8

# Insecticides and Acaricides

| S. No. | Insecticide/ Acaricide | Mode of action | Commercial preparations | Indications | Method of application | Contraindications if any |
|---|---|---|---|---|---|---|
| 1. | **Amidines-Formamidines** | Acts at octapamine receptor sites causing neuronal hyperexcitability and death | Amitraz | Treatment of *Demodex*, *Sarcoptes* and ticks | Spray, dip, pour ons | Contraindicated in horses, pregnant and nursing bitches and cats |
| 2. | **Macrocyclic lactones** | Acts on GABA neurotransmitter | Avermectins, milbemycins, doramectin, eprinomectin, moxidectin, selamectin | endectoparasiticide | Oral, topical-pour ons and spot ons, sub cutaneous injection-lipophilic and is stored in fat tissues and released slowly – metabolized and excreted | In collie breeds and those with mdr gene (multiple drug resistant gene) mutation |

| | | | | | | |
|---|---|---|---|---|---|---|
| 3. | **Carbamates** | Closely related to Organophosphates and are anticholinesterase but unlike OPs appear to cause spontaneously reversible block on enzyme acetylcholinesterase without changing it | Carbaryl, propoxur, fenoxycarb | Used in treatment of ticks lice | Shampoo, topical | --- |
| 4. | **Nitroguanidines** | Chloronicotinyl insecticide, a synthesized chlorinated derivative of nicotine-binds to nicotinic acetylcholine receptors in insects CNS leading to inhibition of cholinergic receptors | Imidacloprid | Used on dogs and cats for flea control | Spot ons | --- |
| 5. | **Organochlorines** | Chlorinated ethanes causes inhibition of sodium conductance along sensory and motor nerve fibres by | DDT, Chlordanes, aldrin, dieldrin, toxaphene, HCH, BHC and Lindane | | | Declined use due to environmental and persistence concerns |

| | | | | | |
|---|---|---|---|---|---|
| | holding the sodium channels open-nerve becomes vulnerable | | | | |
| 6. **Organo-phosphates** | Inhibits the action of acetylcholine esterase at cholinergic synapses at the muscles and plates | Malathion, Sumithion | For insects and arachnids | Can be used in the enviro-ment-sheds etc. | Environ-mental and per-sistence concerns |
| 7. **Phenyl-pyrazoles** | Blocks transmission of signals by inhibitory neurotrans mitter GABA -the compound binds in the chloride channel and inhibits the flux of chloride ion into the nerve cell resulting in hyper excitation of insect nervous system | Fipronil | Sprays/ Spot on-lipophilic and diffuses into the sebaceous gland of hair follicles-residual activity | Pups and kittens for knock down effect on fleas and ticks | |
| 8. **Pyrethrins and synthetic pyrethroids** | Acts on insect CNS by exciting the cell membranes–acts on the sodum channel of the parasite | Perme-thrin, allethrin, delta methrin, flumethrin, cyper-methrin | Lipo-philic, rapidly absorbed, excellent knock down effect, poor | Pour ons, spot ons, spray, dip, topical powder, ear tags | Used with piperonyl butoxide which acts as a synergist |

| | | |
|---|---|---|
| | nerve axons resulting in extended depolarization. synthetic pyrethroids are more stable | residual activity |

# Chapter 9

# Fill Up the Blanks

1. The study of insects is called ........................................... and study of ticks and mites is called ..........................................
2. In general, male insects have .................................................. type of eyes and female insects have ...................................... ................ type of eyes
3. Butchers jelly or Licked beef is a condition caused by the larvae of ..........................................
4. Vomit drops are characteristic of feeding in ....................... ...................
5. Mules operation is a method for control of ............................. ............. in sheep although it is now banned and unethical
6. Based on mouth parts, ticks are classified into .................. ........................ and ..........................................
7. The soft tick which resembles a Guitor or Violin in which adults are non parasitic and nymphs and larvae are parasitic is ..........................................
8. Casting off of the exoskeleton in insects is called ................. ..........................
9. The exoskeleton of insect is in the form of plates or ........................
10. The sclerite on the dorsal aspect is termed the ........................ .................. while that on the ventral aspect is the ......................

.................... and the sclerites on the lateral part of the insect is the ..........................................

11. The two types of metamorphosis are .......................................... and ..........................................
12. Change in form of the insect associated with moulting is termed as ..........................................
13. The jointed leg of insect is made up of pieces called .......................... ................
14. The haemocoel of insect is filled with ..........................................
15. The foregut of insect is termed as ..........................................
16. The posterior hindgut of insect is the..........................................
17. Execretory system of insects includes the ........................... ............... tubules
18. In arachnids .................................. and ...................................... are involved in excretion
19. When compound eyes meet at the midline it is called ..........................................
20. Compound eyes placed far apart are ..........................................
21. The simple eyes are called ..........................................
22. Compound eyes are made up of facets called ........................ ................
23. The organ of Johnston, the auditory organ is present on the ..........................................
24. Antenna covered with hair is .......................................... while that with less hair is called ..........................................
25. Specialized bristle on the third segment of the antenna in Cyclorrhapha is ..........................................
26. .......................................... bears the organ of taste in insects
27. The opening of the salivary gland is in the ........................... ..............
28. Lapping and sponging type of mouth parts is seen in ..........................................

29. Cutting and lapping type of mouth part is characteristic of ..........................................

30. Pipe feeding or feeding from capillary is termed ...........................................

31. Pool feeding as in *Tabanus* sp. is termed ..........................................

32. Sensory pad like structures below the claw of insect is called ..........................................

33. The second pair of wings in Diptera is reduced to form ..........................................

34. The third pair of legs of .......................................... is called the floating legs

35. Wrigglers are .......................................... of mosquitoes while tumblers is the name used to denote the .......................................... stage of mosquitoes

36. Larvae of Culicines are differentiated from Anophelines based on the presence of ..........................................

37. White bands are seen on the joints of legs in the .......................................... mosquito

38. Fishes such as .......................................... are used in control of mosquito

39. .......................................... mosquito larvae are predacious and are used in biological control of other mosquito species.

40. Paris green is the other name for .......................................... used to control mosquito larvae

41. Used in malaria control ITNs are nothing but ..........................................

42. Feathered hairs resembling match stick is characteristic of larvae of ..........................................

43. Indian club shaped larvae is seen in .......................................... nematoceran

44. .......................................... larvae show characteristic eel like movement

45. Crepuscular feeding habit is seen in ...................... nematocera

46. The larvae of .................................... fly has the graber's organ
47. Wings with closed apical cell is seen in .................................... while open apical cell is seen in ..........................................
48. .......................................... fly is a synanthrope
49. .......................................... fly uses vomit drop or the crop fluid to liquefy its food.
50. Both male and female of .......................................... fly suck blood
51. Tarry appearance of the thorax and abdomen is seen in .......................................... adults
52. *Oestrus ovis* lays .......................................... on the nostril of sheep
53. The beef affected by the migration of *Hypoderma lineatum* is called .......................................... while the gelatinous tracks on the beef are termed ..........................................
54. .......................................... and .......................................... are vaccines commercially available against *Rhipicephalus microplus* ticks
55. Intestinal myiasis in horses is caused by ..........................................
56. IGR containing cyromazine commonly used in house fly control is ..........................................
57. Back loss a condition which ends fatally in sheep is due to infestation with ..........................................
58. *Trypanosoma melophagium* is transmitted by .......................... .................
59. .......................................... is the stick tight flea
60. *Xenopsylla cheopsis* is involved in the transmission of .......................................... in humans
61. .......................................... flies are involved in the cyclical transmission of *Trypanosoma theileri.*
62. In sheep, rib cockle is due to heavy infestation with ..........................................
63. Energy for the typical jumping of fleas is stored in rubbery pads of protein called ..........................................

64. 9$^{th}$ abdominal segment of fleas bear a pin cushion like structure on the dorsal aspect which is termed ..........................................

65. The mouth part of bed bugs is of .......................................... type

66. The portion of the idiosoma bearing the legs in arachnids is termed ..........................................

67. The scutum occupies the entire dorsal surface in case of ................................ ixodid ticks whereas in ................................ ixodid ticks scutum occupies the dorsal 1/3 portion alone

68. The function of the gene's organ is application of .................. ...................... on eggs

69. .......................................... stage is non parasitic in *Otobius megnini* tick whereas .......................................... and .................. ...................... stages are parasitic

70. The soft tick that broods over its egg is ..........................................

71. The soft tick generally found in waxy exudates of the ear of livestock is ..........................................

72. An example of a one host tick is ..........................................

73. .................................... ticks complete life cycle using two hosts

74. The toxin .......................................... of *Ixodes holocyclus* is involved in causing tick paralysis

75. *Stylosanthus scabra* has been utilized in the biological control of ..........................................

76. Ticks wave their first pair of legs to identify a potential host, this is termed as ..........................................

77. The portion of the basis capitulum of ticks analogous to antenna of insects is ..........................................

78. .......................................... and .......................................... are burrowing mites while .................................... is a non burrowing mite

79. *Demodex* sp. is seen in .......................................... and .................. ...................... locations

80. .......................................... is used in clearing ticks while mounting them in slides

81. .......................................... solution is used as clearing and mounting medium for mites
82. Skin scrapping is boiled using 10% .......................................... or ..........................................
83. Benzyl phenyl ureas are ..........................................
84. Arthropoda is a greek word meaning ..........................................
85. Exoskeleton of arthropods is made of ..........................................
86. In arthropods, the tergum, sternum and pleuron of each segment are united by more flexible portions of exoskeleton which are termed ..........................................
87. Body cavity of insects is called ..........................................
88. Openings on the wall of heart of insects is called .................. .........................
89. ........................ helps arthropods to orient themselves in space
90. Midgut of insects is called ..........................................
91. The three parts of the digestive system of insects are .................... ........................ , ................................ and ..................................
92. Complete metamorphosis is seen in .......................................... and ..........................................
93. Incomplete metamorphosis is seen in ...................................... , ............................... , ............................ and ..............................
94. In complete metamorphosis the young one is called .......................................... whereas in incomplete metamorphosis the young one is called ..........................................
95. Insect larva with distinct head and mouth parts is called ..........................................
96. Insect larva with reduced head or no head is called ..........................................
97. Insect larva with no thoracic or abdominal legs is called ..........................................
98. Three types of pupa in insects are .......................................... , .......................................... and ..........................................

99. The adult insect inside the pupa is called ........................ ...................

100. The three parts of antenna of insects are .............................. ............ , ..................................... and .....................................

101. Organ of hearing in insects is ......................................... and it is located in the ......................................... segment of antenna

102. Upper lip of insects is called ......................................... and lower lip is called .........................................

103. The three segments in thorax of insects are .............................. ............ , ..................................... and .....................................

104. The parts of legs of insects are ......................................... , ......................................... , ........................................., ......................................... and .........................................

105. In insects, between the claws, a sensory pad like structure or spine/bristle like structure is seen and it is called ......................................... or .........................................

106. ......................................... mosquito rest at an angle to the surface and ......................................... and ......................................... mosquitoes rest parallel to the surface

107. In ......................................... mosquito the maxillary palp is as long as the proboscis and fourth segment is club shaped

108. ......................................... mosquito has short maxillary palp i.e. 1/3rd of the length of proboscis and has pilose antenna

109. ......................................... mosquito is endophilic

110. Pupa of ......................................... mosquito has short and broad breathing trumpets with plamate hairs and spines on all abdominal segments

111. ........................... fly has antenna which projects like two horns

112. Proleg is a feature of larva of .........................................

113. Slipper shaped pupa characterized by cocoon and tuft of respiratory filaments belong to .........................................

114. Terminal abdominal segment of larva of ......................................... has six lobes bearing spines collectively called caudal aster

115. Non retractile forwardly directed baton like proboscis is a feature of ..........................................

116. Larvae of blow flies are called ........................................... or ...........................................

117. Maggots of ..................................... are called surgical maggots

118. Maggots living on wound secrete enzymes which contain uric acid and on oxidation uric acid turns into .................... ...................... which has wound healing properties

119. Field of study where insect stages are used to detect crimes is ...........................................

120. Infestation of live human and vertebrate animals with dipteran larvae which at least for a certain period feed on the host's dead or living tissue, liquid body substances or ingested food is called ...........................................

121. Based on the sequence of egg laying of blow flies myiasis is classified into ......................................... , .................................. and ..........................................

122. Dipteran larvae that require living host for completion of its development is called ..........................................

123. Dipteran larvae that can live on living tissues or as a free living organism either on dead organic matter or on decaying wounds is called ..........................................

124. Based on the area of the body in sheep, strike is classified into .......................................... , .......................................... , .......................................... , .......................................... , .......................................... and ..........................................

125. Nasopharyngeal myiasis or opthalmomyiasis is caused by larvae of ..........................................

126. In sheep, myiasis leads to a condition called ........................ ................. which causes death of affected sheep due to toxaemia and septicaemia

127. .......................................... oil is used to retrieve maggots from myiasis wound

128. ....................... is the winter resting site and .......................... ............ is the spring resting site of *Hypoderma lineatum* in cattle

129. Fly which is active during bright sunny day and has intermittent biting behavior is ..........................................

130. Fly which produces a characteristic noise which leads to avoidance behavior called gadding is .......................................... and this leads to self mutilation

131. Dose of ivermectin is .......................................... and route of administration is ..........................................

132. Fly transmitting pigeon malaria which has strong and spurred claws with crowded veins in wings is ..........................................

133. Hemelytra and ventral thoracic stink glands are features of ..........................................

134. Organ of Ribaga is seen in females of ..........................................

135. .......................................... are wingless insects with laterally compressed bodies which are not strictly host specific

136. Presence of combs or ctenidia are characteristic of .......................................

137. In fleas, adults have .......................................... type of mouth parts and larvae have .......................................... type of mouth parts

138. In .......................................... the third pair of leg is long and powerful adapted for jumping or leaping

139. ............................. flea has a long and slender head with elongate frons with anterior most genal spine as long as the second one

140. ............................. flea has a short and round head with slopy frons with anterior most genal spine shorter than the second one

141. First stage larvae of fleas hatch by cutting through the egg shell with a special tooth called ..........................................

142. In flea bite dermatitis, a hapten in the .................................. of fleas becomes immunogenic by fixation to ................................ in skin

143. MDT stands for ..........................................

144. In fowls stick tight fleas are found mainly in .............................., .......................................... and .................................... regions

145. Nits are eggs of ........................................

146. .......................................... are wingless and dorsoventrally flattened insects which are highly host specific and region specific

147. ........................................ and .......................................... are the two major groups of lice

148. In sucking lice, abdominal segments have dark brown or black areas of thickened chitin known as ........................................

149. Folds present in the posterior margin of the body of ticks is called ........................................

150. Based on ornamentations, ticks are classified into ...................... .................. and .......................................... ticks

151. According to the number of host required by ticks to complete their life cycle, they are classified into ....................................... , ..................................... and ...................................... ticks

152. *Boophilus (Rhipicephalus) microplus* is an example of .................... ...................... host tick

153. *Hyalomma marginatum* is an example of ......................................... host tick

154. *Rhipicephalus sanguineus* is an example of ....................... .................. host tick

155. Soft tick which is oval with slatish blue colour and discs is ........................................

156. First coxa with dorsal hump and ventral notch is a feature of ........................................

157. Hexagonal basis capitulum is found in ................................. tick

158. Spine or Spur in first coxa is a feature in ............................ tick

159. Tick bite is highly painful and annoys the animals and adversely affect the production because of ........................................

160. Tick toxicosis or Sweating sickness in India is mainly caused by .......................................... tick

161. Three types of pheromones which are used in control of ticks are ......................................... , .......................................... and ..........................................

162. Three nymphal stages in mites are .......................................... , .......................................... and ..........................................

163. Larval stages of hard ticks are called ..........................................

164. Tick larvae have .......................................... pairs of legs whereas nymphs and adults have .......................................... pair of legs

165. In unfavourable environment, some species of mites produce nymphs that are adapted to resist adverse conditions called ..........................................

166. Sheep infested with .......................................... demonstrate a nibble reflex characterized by lip smacking and protrusion of the tongue

□□□

Chapter 10

# Multiple Choice Questions

1. Red mange in dogs is caused by

   A. *Sarcoptes scabiei* B. *Otodectes cynotis*

   C. *Demodex canis* D. *Cheyletiella parasitivorax*

2. False Gid/Snotty nose in sheep is caused by the larvae of

   A. *Chrysomyia bezziana* B. *Lucilia cuprina*

   C. *Taenia multiceps* D. *Oestrus ovis*

3. Which of the following is a soft tick

   A. *Ixodes ricinus*

   B. *Argas persicus*

   C. *Hyalomma anatolicum anatolicum*

   D. *Rhipicephalus sanguineus*

4. Moniliform antenna is seen in

   A. *Phlebotomus argentipes* B. *Anopheles stephensi*

   C. *Tabanus striatus* D. *Simulium indicum*

5. Piperonyl butoxide is a
   A. Synthetic pyrethroid
   B. Organophosphate
   C. Synergist used with synthetic pyrethroid
   D. Insect growth regulator

6. *Aedes aegypti* is commonly called
   A. Asian tiger mosquito
   B. The yellow fever mosquito
   C. Dappled mosquito
   D. None of the above

7. Berlese solution is used for
   A. Mounting and clearing insects
   B. Clearing nematodes
   C. Mounting trematodes
   D. Fixing blood smear

8. Diflubenzuron is an example for
   A. Insect growth inhibitor
   B. Insect growth regulator
   C. Juvenile hormone analogue
   D. Synthetic pyrethroid

9. Charles and Miriam Rothschild were associated with
   A. Fleas
   B. Malaria
   C. Filaria
   D. Ticks

10. The only stage of trombiculids which is parasitic is the
    A. Adult
    B. Pupa
    C. Larvae
    D. Nymph

11. Green bottle fly is
    A. *Oestrus ovis*
    B. *Lucilia cuprina*
    C. *Chrysomyia bezziana*
    D. *Sarcophaga ruficornis*

12. Fipronil contains

A. Permethrin
B. Phenylpyrazoles
C. OPs
D. JHA

13. The red mite of poultry is

A. *Ornithonyssus gallinae*
B. *Dermanyssus gallinae*
C. *Cnemidocoptes mutans*
D. *Cnemidocoptes gallinae*

14. An example of a prostriate ticks is

A. *Hyalomma* sp.
B. *Rhipicephalus* sp
C. *Amblyomma* sp.
D. *Ixodes* sp.

15. Queensland itch in horses is caused by

A. *Sarcoptes scabiei*
B. *Simulium* sp.
C. *Demodex* sp.
D. *Culicoides* sp.

16. Stilt like long legs is seen in

A. *Phlebotomus* sp.
B. *Culex* sp.
C. *Tabanus* sp.
D. *Simulium* sp.

17. Seed tick is the

A. Larval stage of hard ticks
B. Nymph of hard tick
C. Protonymph of soft tick
D. Deutonymph of soft tick

18. The yellow body louse of fowl is

A. *Cuclotogaster heterographus*
B. *Menopon gallinae*
C. *Lipeurus caponis*
D. *Menacanthus stramineus*

19. *Haemaphysalis bispinosa* male ticks have

A. Sub anal plates
B. No plates
C. Adanal plates
D. Adanal and accessory adanal plates

20. The tick associated with Kyasanur forest disease is

A. *Hyalomma anatolicum* B. *Haemaphysalis spinigera*

C. *Haemaphysalis bispinosa* D. *Rhipicephalus microplus*

21. Sir. Patrick Manson was associated with the discovery that

A. Malaria was transmitted by mosquitoes

B. Dengue was transmitted by mosquitoes

C. Yellow fever was transmitted by mosquitoes

D. Filarids were transmitted by mosquitoes

22. Crepuscular feeding behaviour is observed in

A. Tabanids B. Ceratopogonids

C. Muscids D. Simulids

23. *Yersina pestis* multiplies in the proventriculus and blocks it in the flea

A. *Ctenocephalides sp.* B. *Pulex sp.*

C. *Spilopsyllus sp.* D. *Xenopsylla* sp.

24. In insects ostia is associated with the

A. Respiratory system B. Reproductive system

C. Circulatory system D. Nervous system

25. The juvenile hormone analogue used in flea control is

A. Cyromazine B. Lufenuron

C. Methoprene D. Pyriproxyfen

26. Velvet mite is the common name of

A. *Sarcoptes scabiei* B. *Trombicula autumnalis*

C. *Cheyletiella yasguri* D. *Otodectes cynotis*

27. TickGARD is a midgut vaccine against

A. *Rhipicephalus sanguineus* B. *Rhipicephalus microplus*

C. *Haemaphysalis bispinosa* D. *Hyalomma marginatum*

28. The type of mouth part of *Musca domestica* is

A. Piercing and sucking type B. Cutting and lapping type

C. Chewing type D. Lapping and sponging type

29. Arista that is bilaterally plumed upto the middle and bare beyond is seen in the case of

A. *Sarcophaga dux* B. *Musca domestica*

C. *Stomoxys calcitrans* D. *Glossina palpalis*

30. *Rhipicephalus microplus* is a

A. Multihost tick B. One host tick

C. Two Host tick D. Three host tick

31. One of the following is not associated with excretion in arthropods

A. Malpighian tubules B. Ostia

C. Coxal gland D. Nephridia

32. The cheek region of insects is referred to as

A. Occiput B. Frons

C. Gena D. Clypeus

33. Sterile insect technique is commonly employed in the control of

A. Ticks B. Mites

C. Blow flies D. Mosquitoes

34. Siphon tube is a feature of larvae of

A. *Anopheles* sp. B. *Phlebotomus* sp.

C. *Simulium* sp. D. *Culex* sp.

35. River blindness in man is due to the bite of infected

A. *Anopheles* sp. B. *Phlebotomus* sp.

C. *Simulium* sp. D. *Culicoides* sp.

36. Fluvial ecosystem/Splash zone is the preferred breeding site for

A. *Anopheles* sp. B. *Phlebotomus* sp.

C. *Simulium* sp. D. *Culicoides sp.*

37. Bird malaria is transmitted by

A. *Culex* sp. B. *Aedes* sp.

C. *Anopheles* sp. D. *Pesudolynchia sp.*

38. Pupa which resembles the head of a ram is characteristic of

A. *Culex* sp. B. *Phlebotomus* sp.

C. *Simulium* sp. D. *Culicoides sp.*

39. The vector for blue tongue in sheep is

A. *Aedes* sp. B. *Phlebotomus* sp.

C. *Triatoma rubrofasciatus* D. *Culicoides sp*

40. The vector for Chikungunya is

A. *Aedes* sp. B. *Anopheles* sp.

C. *Culex* sp. D. *Phlebotomus* sp.

41. Acaricides are used to kill

A. Flies B. Ticks and mites

C. Nematodes D. Protozoa

42. Peritrophic membrane has been used to immunize against

A. *Lucilia* sp. B. *Chrysomyia* sp.

C. *Musca* sp. D. *Anopheles* sp.

43. An example of primary myiasis producer is

A. *Musca domestica* B. *Chrysomyia megacephala*

C. *Lucilia sericata* D. *Sarcophaga dux*

44. Chess board marking on the abdomen is characteristic of

A. *Sarcophaga* sp. B. *Chrysomyia* sp.

C. *Musca* sp. D. *Anopheles* sp

45. Methoprene is a

A. Juvenile hormone analogue

b. Chitin synthesis inhibitor

C. Chitin inhibitor

D. Synthetic pyrethroid

46. *Demodex canis* is seen in

A. Hair follicle B. Cuticle

C. Epidermis D. Skin

47. Benzyl benzoate emulsion is used in the treatment of

A. *Psoroptes ovis* B. *Sarcoptes scabiei*

C. *Demodex canis* D. *Otodectes cynotis*

48. Scutum covers the entire dorsal surface of

A. Ixodid female ticks B. Ixodid male ticks

C. Ixodid larvae D. Ixodid nymphs

49. The portion of the capitulum in ticks used to tear host tissue is

A. Pedipalp B. Hypostome

C. Chelicerae D. Porose area

50. The stage of *Otobius megnini* that is non parasitic

A. Larvae B. Protonymph

C. Deutonymph D. Adult

51. Male ixodid ticks having adanal and accessory adanal plates is characteristic of

A. *Rhipicephalus sanguineus* B. *Rhipicephalus microplus*

C. *Haemaphysalis bispinosa* D. *Hyalomma marginatum*

52. *Theileria annulata* is transmitted transtadially by

A. *Rhipicephalus sanguineus* B. *Rhipicephalus microplus*

C. *Haemaphysalis bispinosa* D. *Hyalomma marginatum*

53. The vector for *Hepatozoon canis* in dogs is

A. *Rhipicephalus sanguineus* B. *Rhipicephalus microplus*

C. *Haemaphysalis bispinosa* D. *Hyalomma marginatum*

54. Castor bean tick is

A. *Amblyomma* sp. B. *Ixodes* sp.

C. *Dermacentor* sp. D. *Hyalomma* sp.

55. Heart water disease in cattle is caused by

A. *Amblyomma* sp. B. *Ixodes* sp.

C. *Dermacentor* sp. D. *Hyalomma* sp.

56. Holocyclotoxin is responsible for

A. Tick toxicosis B. Tick paralysis

C. Bleeding D. Allergy

57. Pustular form of demodicosis is common in

A. Dogs B. Human

C. Cattle D. Cats

58. Miliary dermatitis in cats is associated with infestation with

A. Ticks B. Mites

C. Lice D. Fleas

59. Air breathing organ of terrestrial insects include

    A. Trachea B. Gills

    C. Skin D. Lung books

60. In the male culicidae the mouth parts lack

    A. Mandibles and maxillae B. Labium

    C. Labrum epipharynx D. Hypopharynx

□□□

Chapter 11

# Frequently Asked Subjective Questions

## Short Notes

1. False gid
2. Sweat itch
3. Moulting or Ecdysis in insects
4. Insect growth regulators
5. Tick vaccines
6. Vector potentiality of mosquitoes
7. Soft ticks
8. House fly control
9. Types of insect pupa
10. Sheep ked
11. Butchers jelly or Licked beef
12. Gastric myiasis in horses
13. Lice infestation in poultry
14. Stick tight flea
15. Types of insect larva
16. Differences between complete and incomplete metamorphosis

17. Biological control of ticks
18. Fowl tick
19. Tick paralysis
20. Red mite of poultry
21. Processing of skin scrapping
22. Forest fly
23. Mouth parts of *Musca domestica*
24. Depluming itch
25. Nasal bot fly
26. Nasal myiasis
27. Pheromone based control of flies and ticks
28. Heel fly
29. Write about the lifecycle and effect on host of *Simulium* sp.
30. Bed bugs
31. Control of lice infestation in poultry
32. IGR
33. Spinose ear tick
34. Vaccines against ticks
35. Novel methods of mosquito control
36. *Simulium*
37. Habits and control of *Culicoides sp.*
38. Owl midges
39. Mode of feeding of *Tabanus* and its implication on disease transmission
40. Flesh fly
41. Oriental rat flea
42. Insect collection and preservation
43. Adult immersion test

44. Larval packet test
45. Flea allergic dermatitis
46. Exoskeleton
47. Synthetic pyrethroids
48. Blow flies classification
49. Collection and processing of ticks
50. Adaptation to parasitic life by fleas

## Essay

1. Define "Myiasis". Write in detail about classification, pathogenesis, treatment and control of Myiasis in sheep
2. List out the hard ticks affecting livestock. Discuss the treatment and control of ticks with emphasis on tick vaccines
3. Describe in detail about Sarcoptic mange
4. Compare between the family Sarcoptidae and Psoroptidae and write briefly on the burrowing mite
5. Describe in detail demodicosis in dogs
6. Describe the Morphology, lifecycle, effect on the host of the brachyceran fly
7. Enlist the bot flies affecting livestock and give an account of the sheep nasal bot fly.
8. Enumerate the flies affecting livestock and write briefly on the common house fly its economic impact and control measures
9. Compare the different nematocerans morphologically and write how you will control them
10. Name the fleas affecting animals and write about the new methods employed in their control
11. Discuss in detail the insecticides used in the control of flies of veterinary importance
12. Differentiate between Argasidae and Ixodidae
13. Give an account of the ox warble fly

14. Differentiate between Anopheline and Culicine mosquitoes
15. Draw the mouth parts of house fly and label the parts. How does the feeding process help in transmitting diseases
16. Write about the effect of ticks on the host, problems related to resistance and how to overcome them
17. What is acaricide resistance? Explain how the FAO prescribed tests to detect acaricide resistance are conducted
18. Give an account of *Hypoderma lineatum*
19. List the insecticides and acaricides used in livestock with their mode of action
20. Describe the various methods of application of insecticides and acaricides to livestock and poultry

□□□

Chapter 12

# Important Text Books in Veterinary Entomology and Acarology


1. Veterinary Entomology - Richard Wall and David Shearer (London, Chapman and Hall, 1997)
2. Medical and Veterinary Entomology - Garry R. Mullen and Lance A. Durden
3. Medical and Veterinary Entomology - D.S. Kettle
4. Helminths, Arthropods and Protozoa of domesticated animals: EJL Soulsby


□□□

Chapter 13

# Answers - Fill Up the Blanks

1. Entomology, Acarology
2. holoptic, dichoptic
3. *Hypoderma* sp.
4. *Musca domestica*
5. Myiasis
6. longirostrate, brevirostrate
7. *Otobius megnini*
8. Moulting or Ecdysis
9. Sclerites
10. Tergum, Sternum, Pleuron
11. Complete (Holometabola) and Incomplete (Hemimetabola)
12. Metamorphosis
13. Podomeres
14. Haemolymph
15. Stomodaeum
16. Proctodaeum
17. Malpighian tubules

18. Coxal glands and Malpighian tubules
19. Holoptic
20 Dichoptic
21. Ocelli
22. Ommatidia
23. Second segment of antenna (Pedicel)
24. Plumose, pilose
25. Arista
26. Epipharynx
27. Hypopharynx
28. *Musca domestica*
29. *Tabanus*
30. Solenophagy
31. Telmophagy
32. Pulvillus
33. Halteres or Balancers
34. Mosquito
35. Larva, pupa
36. Siphon tube
37. *Aedes* sp.
38. *Gambusia sp*
39. *Toxorhynchites sp*
40. Copper acetoarsenite
41. Insecticide treated bed nets
42. *Phlebotomus sp*
43. *Simulium sp*
44. *Culicoides sp*
45. *Culicoides sp*

46. *Tabanus striatus*
47. *Musca domestica, Stomoxys calcitrans*
48. *Musca domestica*
49. *Musca domestica*
50. *Stomoxys calcitrans*
51. *Oestrus ovis*
52. Larvae
53. Licked beef, butchers jelly
54. Tickgard, Gavac
55. *Gasterophilus equi*
56. Larvadex
57. Sheep ked
58. *Melophagus ovinus* / Sheep ked
59. *Echidnophaga gallinacea*
60. Plague/*Yersinia pestis*
61. *Hippobosca sp*
62. *Melophagus ovinus*
63. Resilin
64. Sensilium/Pygidium
65. Piercing and sucking
66. Podosoma
67. Male, female
68. Wax
69. Adult, larvae, nymphs
70. *Ornithodoros savignyi*
71. *Otobius megnini*
72. *Boophilus (Rhipicephalus) microplus*
73. Two host tick

74. Holocyclotoxin
75. Ticks
76. Questing
77. Pedipalp
78. *Sarcoptes scabiei, Demodex canis, Psoroptes ovis*
79. Hair follicles, sebaceous glands
80. Carbolic acid
81. Berlese solution
82. KOH or NaOH
83. Chitin synthesis inhibitors/IGRs
84. Jointed legs
85. Chitin
86. Sutures
87. Haemocoel
88. Ostia
89. Statocysts
90. Mesenteron
91. Foregut, midgut and hindgut
92. Flies, fleas
93. Ticks, lice, mites, bugs
94. Larva, nymph
95. Eucephalus
96. Acephalus
97. Apodous
98. Exarate (free), obtectate, coarctate
99. Imago
100. Scape, pedicel, flagellum
101. Organ of Johnston, second

102. Labrum, labium
103. Prothorax, mesothorax and metathorax
104. Coxa, trochanter, femur, tibia, tarsus
105. Empodium, arolium
106. *Anopheles sp., Culex sp., Aedes sp.*
107. Male *Anopheles sp.*
108. Female *Culex sp.*
109. *Aedes sp.*
110. *Anopheles sp.*
111. *Simulium sp.*
112. *Simulium sp.*
113. *Simulium sp.*
114. *Tabanus sp.*
115. *Stomoxys calcitrans*
116. Screw worms or maggots
117. *Chrysomyia sp.*
118. Allantoin
119. Forensic entomology
120. Myiasis
121. Primary, secondary and tertiary
122. Obligatory
123. Facultative
124. Breech strike or crutch strike, tail strike, pizzle strike, poll strike, body strike and wound strike
125. *Oestrus ovis*
126. Lightning strike
127. Turpentine
128. Connective tissue of oesophageal wall, subcutaneous tissue of the back

129. *Tabanus striatus*
130. *Tabanus striatus*
131. 200 μg or 0.2 mg/kg body wt, subcutaneous
132. *Pseudolynchia canariensis*
133. *Cimex sp.*
134. *Cimex sp*
135. Fleas
136. Fleas
137. Piercing and sucking, mastigatory
138. Fleas
139. *Ctenocephalides felis*
140. *Ctenocephalides canis*
141. Egg tooth
142. Saliva, collagen
143. Maggot debridement therapy
144. Comb, wattles and around eyes
145. Lice
146. Lice
147. Biting lice and sucking lice
148. Paratergal plates
149. Festoons
150. Ornate, inornate
151. One host, two host, three host
152. One
153. Two
154. Three
155. *Argas persicus*
156. *Boophilus sp.*

157. *Rhipicephalus sanguineus*
158. *Haemaphysalis sp.*
159. Tick worry
160. *Hyalomma truncatum*
161. Assembly pheromone, aggregation and attachment pheromone, sex pheromone
162. Protonymph, deutonymph, tritonymph
163. Seed ticks
164. Three, four
165. Hypopial nymphs or hypopi
166. Sheep scab

## Multiple choice questions

|  |  |
|---|---|
| 1. C | 2. D |
| 3. B | 4. A |
| 5. C | 6. A |
| 7. A | 8. B |
| 9. A | 10. C |
| 11. B | 12. B |
| 13. B | 14. D |
| 15. D | 16. A |
| 17. A | 18. D |
| 19. B | 20. B |
| 21. D | 22. B |
| 23. D | 24. C |
| 25. C | 26. B |
| 27. B | 28. D |
| 29. A | 30. B |
| 31. B | 32. C |

33. C
34. D
35. C
36. C
37. A
38. B
39. D
40. A
41. B
42. A
43. C
44. A
45. A
46. A
47. B
48. B
49. C
50. D
51. D
52. D
53. A
54. B
55. A
56. B
57. C
58. D
59. A
60. A

□□□

# PART-III

# VETERINARY PROTOZOOLOGY

Chapter 1

# Common Name of Diseases and Causative Protozoa

| S.No. | Name of the disease/ condition | Causative Protozoa |
|---|---|---|
| 1. | Surra- in all hosts | *Trypanosoma evansi* |
| | In horses-Derrengadara, Nikhalgaya, Dubli, Murrina, Mal de caderas | |
| | In camels- Tibersa (Three year disease), El dembori, Purana, Gufar or Dioufar | |
| | In elephants-Thut | |
| 2. | Dourine in horses/covering disease/breeding paralysis | *Trypanosoma equiperdum* |
| 3. | Paranagana, Gambia fever, Ghindi and Gobial | *Trypanosoma congolense* |
| 4. | Nagana | *Trypanosoma congolense, Trypanosma brucei* |
| 5. | Souma | *Trypanosma vivax* |
| 6. | American human trypanosomosis, Chagas disease | *Trypanosoma cruzi* |
| 7. | Gambian sleeping sickness, Chronic sleeping sickness of man | *Trypanosoma gambiense* |

| | | |
|---|---|---|
| 8. | East African sleeping sickness, Acute sleeping sickness | *Trypanosoma rhodesiense* |
| 9. | Visceral leishmaniosis, Kala azar, Dum dum fever, Black fever, Infantile splenomegaly, Tropical splenomegaly, Death sickness, Spleenic fever | *Leishmania donovani* |
| 8. | Cutaneous leishmaniasis, Old world cutaneous leishmaniasis, Oriental sore, Aleppo button, Delhi boil, Jericho boil. Dry or Urban cutaneous leishmaniasis, Tropical ulcer | *Leishmania tropica* |
| 9. | Moist or Rural cutaneous leishmaniasis, Muco cutaneous leishmaniasis | *Leishmania tropica major* |
| 10. | Espundia | *Leishmania braziliensis* |
| 11. | Uta | *Leishmania peruviana* |
| 12. | Chiclero ulcer, Bay sore | *Leishmania mexicana mexicana* |
| 12. | Infectious enterohepatitis in turkey, Black head disease, Histomonosis, Typhlohepatitis | *Histomonas meleagridis* |
| 13. | Pigeon Canker, Upper digestive tract trichomonosis, Avian trichomonosis in pigeons, Frounce in falcons/ yellow button | *Trichomonas gallinae* |
| 14. | Bovine trichomonosis, Bovine venereal disease | *Tritrichomonas foetus* |
| 15. | Traveler's diarrhea, Beaver fever, Giardiosis, Lambliosis | *Giardia lamblia* |
| 16. | Amoebiasis, Amoebic dysentery, Amoebic liver abscess, Hepatic or extraintestinal amoebosis, Amoebic granuloma, Gut perforation | *Entamoeba histolytica* |

| | | |
|---|---|---|
| 17. | Caecal coccidiosis of poultry | *Eimeria tenella* |
| 18. | Intestinal coccidiosis of poultry | *Eimeria necatrix* |
| 19. | Rectal coccidiosis of poultry | *Eimeria brunetti* |
| 20. | Winter coccidiosis in cattle, Red dysentery in cattle | *Eimeria zuernii* |
| 21. | Abortion storm in sheep, Toxoplasmosis | *Toxoplasma gondii* |
| 22. | Pigeon malaria | *Haemoproteus columbae* |
| 23. | Cattle tick fever, Texas fever, Red water fever, Piroplasmosis | *Babesia bigemina* |
| 24. | Canine babesiosis, Biliary fever, Malignant jaundice, Nambiuvu (Bloody ears) | *Babesia canis* |
| 25. | Tropical bovine theileriosis, Tropical piroplasmosis, Egyptian fever, Mediterranean fever | *Theileria annulata* |
| 26. | Benign bovine theileriosis, Tzaneen disease, Marica calf disease, Mild gall sickness | *Theileria mutans* |
| 27. | Fowl malaria, Avian malaria | *Plasmodium gallinaceum* |
| 28. | Cryptosporidiosis | *Cryptosporidium parvum* |
| 29. | Isosporosis | *Isospora felis, Isospora canis* |
| 30. | Sarcocystosis, Dalmeny disease | *Sarcocystis cruzi* |
| 31. | Neosporosis | *Neospora caninum* |
| 32. | Hepatozoonosis | *Hepatozoon canis* |
| 33. | Anaplasmosis, Gall sickness | *Anaplasma marginale, Anaplasma centrale* |
| 34. | Canine ehrlichiosis, Tropical canine pancytopenia, Tracker dog disease, Lahore disease, Nairobi bleeding disease | *Ehrlichia canis* |

| | | |
|---|---|---|
| 35. | East Coast Fever, Corridor's disease, Turning sickness | *Theileria parva* |
| 36. | Balantidosis | *Balantidium coli* |
| 37. | Cerebral babesiosis in cattle | *Babesia bovis* |
| 38. | Cerebral babesiosis in dog | *Babesia canis* |
| 39. | Equine babesiosis | *Theileria equi, Babesia caballi* |
| 40. | Bovine ehrlichiosis, NOFEL, NOPI | *Ehrlichia bovis* |
| 41. | Leucocytozoonosis, Bangkok haemorrhagic disease | *Leucocytozoon caulleryi* or *Akiba caulleryi* |
| 42. | Malignant ovine and caprine theileriosis | *Theileria lestoquardi* |
| 43. | Potomac horse fever | *Ehrlichia equi* |

❑❑❑

Chapter 2

# Protozoa and Their Vectors

| S.No. | Protozoa | Vector |
|---|---|---|
| 1. | *Trypanosoma evansi* | *Tabanus, Haematopota, Stomoxys* |
| 2. | *Trypanosoma theileri* | *Hippobosca, Tabanus* |
| 3. | *Trypanosoma congolense* | *Glossina sp.* |
| 4. | *Trypanosoma vivax* | *Glossina sp.* |
| 5. | *Trypanosoma brucei* | *Glossina sp.* |
| 6. | *Leishmania donovani* | *Phlebotomus argentipes* |
| 7. | *Leishmania tropica* | *Phlebotomus sergenti* |
| 8. | *Plasmodium gallinaceum* | *Mansonia* sp., *Armigeres* sp., *Culex sp., Aedes sp.* of mosquitoes |
| 9. | *Haemoproteus columbae* | *Pseudolynchia canariensis* |
| 10. | *Babesia bigemina* | *Rhipicephalus microplus, R. annulatus* |
| 11. | *Babesia bovis* | *Rhipicephalus microplus, R.annulatus* |
| 12. | *Babesia caballi* | *Dermacenter sp, Hyalomma excavatum, H.dromedarii, Rhipicephalus bursa, R.sanguineus* |
| 13. | *Babesia motasi* | *Rhipicephalus bursa, Dermacenter sylvarum, Haemaphysalis punctata* |
| 14. | *Babesia ovis* | *Rhipicephalus bursa* |

| | | |
|---|---|---|
| 15. | *Babesia canis* | *Rhipicephalus sanguineus* |
| 16. | *Babesia gibsoni* | *Rhipicephalus sanguineus, Haemaphysalis bispinosa* |
| 17. | *Theileria annulata* | *Hyalomma anatolicum anatolicum, Hyalomma marginatum isaaci* |
| 18. | *Theileria equi* | *Hyalomma excavatum, H.dromoderi, Rhipicephalus bursa, R.dronicus, R.sanguineus* |
| 19. | *Theileria parva* | *Rhipicephalus appendiculatus, R.evertsi, Hyalomma excavatum, H. dromadari, H. truncatum* |
| 20. | *Hepatozoon canis* | *Rhipicephalus sanguineus* |
| 21. | *Ehrlichia canis* | *Rhipicephalus sanguineus* |
| 22. | *Trypanosoma cruzi* | Reduvid bug/Kissing bug/Cone nosed bug/Triatoma bug of *Triatoma, Rhodnius,* and *Panstrongylus* genera |
| 23. | *Plasmodium falciparum* | *Anopheles sp.* |
| 24. | *Leucocytozoon caulleryi* | *Culicoides sp.* |
| 25. | *Anaplasma marginale* and *Anaplasma centrale* | *Hyalomma sp., Haemaphysalis sp., Boophilus (Rhipicephalus) sp.* |

□□□

Chapter 3

# Morphological Characteristics of Protozoa

| S.No. | Protozoa | Description |
|---|---|---|
| 1. | *Trypanosoma evansi* | Seen outside blood cells |
| | | Leaf like |
| | | Flagellum present |
| | | Undulating membrane present |
| 2. | *Babesia bigemina* | Found inside RBC |
| | | Pear shaped |
| | | Seen as pairs |
| 3. | *Babesia canis* | Found inside RBC |
| | | Pear shaped |
| | | Seen as pairs although multiple infections are common (>16 organisms in single RBC) |
| 4. | *Theileria annulata* (Piroplasm) | Found inside RBC |
| | | Round or oval or ring forms or rod or comma shaped |
| 5. | *Theileria annulata* (Schizont or Koch's blue bodies) | Found inside lymphocytes |
| | | Circular or irregular shape |
| 6. | *Ehrlichia canis* | Found inside monocytes |
| | | Morula forms seen |

| | | |
|---|---|---|
| 7. | *Anaplasma marginale* | Found inside RBC |
| | | In margin of RBC seen as dots surrounded by a halo |
| 8. | *Haemporoteus columbae* | Halter or sausage shaped gamonts found inside RBC |
| 9. | *Plasmodium gallinaceum* | Gamonts or segmenter found inside RBC |
| 10. | *Hepatozoon canis* | Gelatin capsule shaped gamonts inside Neutrophil |
| 11. | *Trypanosoma theileri* | Large size (60-70 µm up to 120 µm) |
| | | Posterior end is long and pointed |
| | | Well developed undulating membrane |
| | | Well defined free flagellum |
| 12. | *Leishmania* amastigotes | Small spherical or ovoid |
| | | Red oval nucleus and bluish cytoplasm |
| | | Visible nucleus and kinetoplast |
| 13. | *Leishmania* promastigotes | Spindle shaped |
| | | Free flagellum as long as the body |
| | | No undulating membrane |
| 14. | *Trichomonas gallinae* | Pyriform shaped |
| | | Four anterior flagella |
| | | Crescent shaped pelta |
| | | Narrow axostyle |
| | | Undulating membrane up to 3/4th of the body |
| | | No free flagellum |
| 15. | *Giardia lamblia* trophozoites | Bilaterally symmetrical |
| | | Pear or ellipsoidal shape |
| | | Adhesive disc present |
| | | Eight flagella in four rows |
| | | Resemble "Monkey face" or "Smiley face" |

| | | |
|---|---|---|
| 16. | *Giardia lamblia* cyst | Ovoid in shape<br>Thin cyst wall<br>Two to four nuclei with prominent comma shaped bodies<br>Mature cyst has four nuclei |
| 17. | *Entamoeba histolytica* trophozoite | Granular endoplasm and hyaline ectoplasm<br>Presence of pseudopodia<br>Single spherical nucleus with endosome<br>Presence of food vacuoles |
| 18. | *Entamoeba histolytica* cyst | Spherical to ovoid<br>Cyst wall is present<br>Presence of chromatoid bodies<br>Mature cyst is quadrinucleate |
| 19. | *Eimeria* unsporulated oocyst | Oval or Spherical<br>Two layered oocyst wall<br>Undifferentiated mass "sporont" inside |
| 20. | *Eimeria* sporulated oocyst | Oval or Spherical<br>Two layered oocyst wall<br>Presence of four sporocysts each containing two sporozoites inside |
| 21. | *Isospora* sporulated oocyst | Oval<br>Single layered oocyst wall<br>Presence of two sporocysts each containing four sporozoites inside |
| 22. | *Toxoplasma gondii* tachyzoites | Arc or Crescent shaped<br>Central nucleus |
| 23. | *Toxoplasma gondii* bradyzoites | Cyst size is 100 µm<br>It contains about 60,000 lancet shaped tightly packed bradyzoites inside |

| | | |
|---|---|---|
| 24. | *Sarcocystis tenella* muscle section | Seen in striated muscles<br>Cylindrical or spindle shape<br>Cyst wall present<br>Meischer's tubules present inside |
| 25. | *Balantidium coli* trophozoite | Ovoid shape<br>Body covered with cilia<br>Sausage shaped macronucleus and small micronucleus<br>Presence of cytopyge<br>Food vacuoles and contractile vacuoles present |
| 26. | *Neospora caninum* oocyst | Smooth wall<br>No micropyle<br>Contains two sporocysts each containing four sporozoites |
| 27. | *Cryptosporidium* oocyst | Spherical shape<br>Contains four naked sporozoites |
| 28. | *Histomonas* in liver section | Seen in clusters or singly<br>Amoeboid nature<br>Flagella absent |

□□□

Chapter 4

# Diagnosis of Protozoa

| S.No. | Protozoa | Material to be taken for diagnosis/ Specific diagnostic tests/Culture media |
|---|---|---|
| 1 | *Theileria annulata* | Lymph node biopsy, blood smear |
| 2. | *Babesia sp.* | Peripheral blood smears |
| 3. | *Hepatozoon canis* | Buffy coat smear, blood smear |
| 4. | *Haemoproteus columbae* | Blood smear |
| 5. | Coccidiosis | Faeces/dung, in case of PM examination collect intestine for developmental stages, Oocyst coproculture using 2.5% potassium dichromate, Lesion scoring method |
| 6. | *Trypanosoma* | Wet film examination or Direct examination of blood film, thick/thin blood smear examination, Buffy coat smear examination, Microhaematocrit<br>Animal inoculation in rat, mice and guinea pigs<br>Culture in RPMI 1640<br>Non specific chemical tests like Mercurric chloride test, Stilbamidine test, Formal gel test and Nitric acid test |
| 7. | *Leishmania donovani* | Sternal biopsy or iliac lymph node biopsy |

| | | |
|---|---|---|
| | | Crest puncture for taking bone marrow or spleen biopsy, peripheral blood smear or thick smear, culture of blood in NNN media |
| 8. | *Leishmania tropica* | Smears from the periphery of the cutaneous lesion, proximal lymph node biopsy, culture in NNN medium |
| 9. | *Trichomonas gallinae* | Throat swab examination |
| 10. | *Tritrichomonas foetus* | Examination of preputial washing, vaginal, mucopurulent discharge from uterus, Cervical mucus agglutination test, Culture in CPLM (cysteine-peptone liver extract maltose serum) BGPS (beef extract glucose, peptone serum) (or) Diamond's media, Intradermal test |
| 11. | *Toxoplasma gondii* | Cerebrospinal fluid examination, Sabin Feldman Dye test, Tissue biopsy |
| 12. | *Entamoeba histolytica* | Schaudinn haematoxylin staining technique, Heidenhain's iron haematoxylin- faecal smears, identification of cysts by ZnSO4 floatation, formalin triton ether and merthiolate iodine formaldehyde concentration methods |
| 13. | *Cryptosporidium parvum* | Modified Ziehl-Nielsen's staining of faecal smear/Acid fast staining, Carbol fuchsin staining, Sheather's sugar/Zinc sulphate floatation, formalin-ether concentration, and formalin-ethylacetate sedimentation to concentrate oocysts |
| 14. | *Trypanosoma cruzi* | Xenodiagnosis, Strout technique, Microhaematocrit |
| 15. | *Plasmodium gallinaceum* | Blood smear |
| 16. | *Anaplasma sp.* | Blood smear |
| 17. | *Ehrlichia sp.* | Blood smear |
| 18. | *Giardia lamblia* | Identification of cysts by ZnSO4 floatation |

- All protozoans can be detected by Polymerase chain reaction (PCR)

Chapter 5

# Protozoan Stages – Location and Hosts

| S. No. | Protozoa | Stage and Definitive host(s) | Location | Stage and Intermediate host(s) | Location |
|---|---|---|---|---|---|
| 1. | *Trypanosoma evansi* | **Trypomastigote** Horse, cattle, buffalo, camel, dog and in wild animals viz. Lion, Tiger, leopard, elephant rarely in sheep, goats, cat and pig | Blood stream as extracellular and in tissue fluids | --- | --- |
| 2. | *Trypanosoma theileri* | **Trypomastigote and Epimastigote** Domestic cattle, buffaloes, zebu, bison, antelope, deer | Blood and lymph | --- | --- |
| 3. | *Trypanosoma brucei* | **Trypomastigote** Horse, | Blood | --- | --- |

| | | | | | |
|---|---|---|---|---|---|
| | | Donkey, Ox, Sheep, Goat etc. | | | |
| 4. | *Trypanosoma vivax* | **Trypoma-stigote** Cattle, Buffalo, Sheep, Goat, Camel and Horses | Blood | --- | --- |
| 5. | *Trypanosoma congolense* | **Trypoma-stigote** Cattle, Sheep, goats, Pigs and Horses | Blood | --- | --- |
| 6. | *Trypanosoma equiperdum* | Horse | Cutaneous and genital lesions | --- | --- |
| 7. | *Trypanosoma cruzi* | **Trypoma-stigote** Human beings chiefly children and infants | Mainly Intracellular in reticulo-endothelial cells and also in blood | --- | --- |
| 8. | *Trypanosoma gambiense* | **Trypoma-stigote** Human beings | Blood | --- | --- |
| 9. | *Trypanosoma rhodesiense* | **Trypoma-stigote** Human beings | Blood | --- | --- |
| 10. | *Leishmania donovani* | **Amastigote** Human beings | Cells of the reticulo-endothelial system of spleen, liver, bone marrow and lymph node | --- | --- |
| 11. | *Leishmania tropica* | **Amastigote** Human beings and dog ***Rodents act** | Skin | --- | --- |

| | | | | | |
|---|---|---|---|---|---|
| | | **as reservoir hosts** | | | |
| 12. | *Tritri-chomonas foetus* | Cattle, occasionally in buffaloes, possibly in pig, horse, deer, sheep and rodents | Bull - Preputial cavity/ sheath, urethra Cow - Vagina, cervix, uterus, foetus | --- | --- |
| 13. | *Trichomonas gallinae* | Pigeon, turkey, chicken | Upper digestive tract-crop, mouth, palate and up to proventri-culus/rarely in liver | --- | --- |
| 14. | *Histomonas meleagridis* | Turkeys, chicken, guinea fowl and other birds | Caeca, liver | --- | --- |
| 15. | *Giardia lamblia* | **Trophozoite** Man and non human primates (Monkeys, Gorilla, Chimpanzee), possibly in pig, dog, cat and other animals<br>Cysts are voided in the faeces and disease spreads via faeco-oral contami-nation | Duodenum, upper ileum and colon | --- | --- |

| | | | | | |
|---|---|---|---|---|---|
| 16. | *Entamoeba histolytica* | **Trophozoite** Man, chimpanzees (**Zooanthroponotic disease**) Dogs, pig, cat, swine, cattle – rare<br>Cysts are voided in the faeces and disease spreads via faeco-oral contamination | Large intestine especially the ileo-caecal junction and sigmoido-colon<br>Extra intestinally in liver, lung, brain, spleen and subcutaneous tissue | --- | --- |
| 17. | *Eimeria tenella* | Domestic fowl | Caecum (Schizogony and gametogonic cycles occur in caecum) | --- | --- |
| 18. | *Eimeria necatrix* | Domestic fowl | Small intestine and Caecum (Schizogony in mid small intestine and gametogony in caecum) | --- | --- |
| 19. | *Eimeria maxima* | Domestic fowl | Small intestine | --- | --- |
| 20. | *Eimeria acervulina* | Domestic fowl | Duodenum | --- | --- |
| 21. | *Eimeria brunetti* | Domestic fowl | Rectum | --- | --- |
| 22. | *Eimeria zuernii* | Cattle, zebu, water buffalo | Small intestine and large intestine<br>(caecum, | --- | --- |

| | | | | | |
|---|---|---|---|---|---|
| | | | colon and rectum) | | |
| 23. | *Eimeria bovis* | Cattle, zebu, water buffalo | Small intestine and terminal part of ileum, caecum and colon<br>Schizogony in small intestine and gametogony in terminal part of ileum, caecum and colon | --- | --- |
| 24. | *Eimeria ninakohlya-kimovae* | Sheep | Ileum, caecum and colon | --- | --- |
| 25. | *Eimeria arloingi* | Goat | Small intestine | --- | --- |
| 26. | *Isospora felis* | Domestic cat, Wild cat, Tiger , Lion | Small intestine, caecum, occasionally in colon | --- | --- |
| 27. | *Toxoplasma gondii* | **Meronts, gamonts, oocyst** Domestic cat, Jaguarundi, Ocelot, Leopard cat | Small intestine - Epithelial cells of villi | **Meronts and merozoites (tachyzoite)** Warm blooded animals including man, domestic animals, wild animals, birds. Over 200 species are reported as intermediate host | Neurons, microglia, endothelium of liver, parenchymal cells, lung, cardiac, skeletal muscle, foetal membrane, macrophages, leucocytes. In acute infection merozoites (tachyzoite) are free in blood and peritoneal exudate |

| | | | | | |
|---|---|---|---|---|---|
| 28. | *Sarcocystis cruzi* | **Gamonts and oocysts** Dogs, wolves, coyotes, racoons, foxes, hyenas | Intestinal epithelial cells | **Tachyzoite and Bradyzoite (Sarcocyst)** cattle, sheep, goat, pig, horse, rabbit, chicken and man | Vascular endothelium of visceral organs and muscular and neural tissues |
| 29. | *Neospora caninum* | Dogs | Small intestine | **Tissue cyst** Cattle | Tissues |
| 30. | *Cryptosporidium parvum* | Cattle, man Oocysts are voided in the faeces and disease spreads via faeco-oral contamination | Small and Large intestine | --- | --- |
| 31. | *Plasmodium gallinaceum* | **Gamonts** Birds | RBC | --- | --- |
| 32. | *Haemoproteus columbae* | **Gamonts** Domestic and wild pigeons, Mourning doves, Turtle doves and number of wild birds | RBC | --- | --- |
| 33. | *Babesia bigemina* | **Merozoites** Cattle and Buffaloes | RBC | --- | --- |
| 34. | *Babesia bovis* | **Merozoites** Cattle and Buffaloes | RBC | --- | --- |
| 34. | *Babesia canis* | **Merozoites** Domestic dog, Wolf, Coyote, Jackal, Fox | RBC | --- | --- |

| | | | | | |
|---|---|---|---|---|---|
| 35. | *Babesia gibsoni* | **Merozoites** Domestic dog, jackal, wolf, Indian wild dog, fox<br>Jackal is the natural host in India | RBC | --- | --- |
| 36. | *Theileria annulata* | Bovine, Zebu, and water buffalo | RBC-Piroplasm Lymphocyte-Schizont (Koch's blue bodies) | --- | --- |
| 37. | *Theileria hirci* | Sheep and goats | RBC-Piroplasm Lymphocyte-Schizont (Koch's blue bodies) | --- | --- |
| 38. | *Balantidium coli* | **Trophozoite** Pig, man, chimpanzee, Rhesus monkey, guinea pig, rarely in dog and rat<br>Cysts are voided in the faeces and disease spreads via faeco-oral contamination | Colon | --- | --- |
| 39. | *Anaplasma marginale* | Cattle, Deer, Sheep, Goats, Buffalo, Camel, Antelope, Zebra | RBC (margin) | --- | --- |

| | | | | | |
|---|---|---|---|---|---|
| 40. | *Anaplasma centrale* | Cattle, Deer, Sheep, Goats, Buffalo, Camel, Antelope, Zebra | RBC (centre) | --- | --- |
| 41. | *Ehrlichia canis* | **Morula** Canines | Monocyte | --- | --- |
| 42. | *Ehrlichia bovis* | **Morula** Bovines | Monocyte | --- | --- |
| 43. | *Ehrlichia equi* | **Morula** Horse | Monocyte | --- | --- |
| 44. | *Hepatozoon canis* | **Gamonts** Dog | Neutrophil | --- | --- |
| 45. | *Leucocytozoon caulleryi* | **Gamonts** Chicken, Guinea fowls | RBC | --- | --- |

□□□

Chapter 6

# Antiprotozoal Drugs

| S.No. | Disease | Drug | Dose | Route |
|---|---|---|---|---|
| 1. | Trypano-somosis | Diminazine aceturate | Cattle, Horse, Sheep 0.8-1.6g/100kg<br>Dog: 3.5- 7 mg/kg<br>Two doses | I/M |
| | | Antrycide-methyl sulphate (Quinapyra-mine dimethyl sulphate)<br>10% solution in water | 5 mg/kg | S/C |
| | | Antrycide prosalt (Antrycide chloride and Antrycide sulphate in 3:2 ratio)<br>Curative and Prophylactic drug | 7.4 mg/kg | S/C |
| | | Suramin | 4 g/ 45 kg | I/V |
| | | | Dogs: 0.3 g for 6 days | I/V |
| | | Homidium bromide & Homidium chloride | 1.25 mg/kg single dose | I/M |
| | | Pyrithidium bromide-4% | 2 mg/kg | S/C |

| | | | | |
|---|---|---|---|---|
| 2. | Visceral Leish-maniosis | Pentamidine isethionate | 4 mg/kg – 10 days, 3 courses- Dog | I/M |
| | | Pentavalent antimony sodium gluconate | 400 mg daily for children and 600 mg daily for adults - 6-30 days | I/M or I/V |
| | | Sodium stibo gluconate | 20 mg/kg/day (Max: 850 mg/day) | Slow I/V |
| | | Amphotericin B | 1 mg/kg – 0.01% in 5% dextrose for 45 days to 8 weeks | I/V |
| | | Meglumine antimoniate | 30-50 mg/kg/day for 10-12 days | I/V |
| 3. | Cutaneous Leish-maniosis | Sodium stibo gluconate | Double the dose for that of Visceral Leishmaniosis | |
| | | Amphotericin B | Double the dose for that of Visceral Leishmaniosis | |
| | | Quinacrine HCl | 200 mg at the base of ulcer | Topical |
| 4. | Bovine tricho-monosis (Bulls) | Diminazine aceturate-1% solution | 100-150 ml – 5 treatments | Injected into prepuce |
| | | Acriflavin | 1% soln or ointment | Massage into the prepuce |
| | | Dimetridazole | 50 mg/kg – daily for 5 days | Oral |
| | | | 10 mg/kg for 5 days | I/V |
| | | Hydrogen peroxide | 3% | Preputial wash |
| 5. | Bovine trichomono-sis (Cows) | Metronidazole | 66 mg/kg thrice daily for 5 days | |
| 6. | Trichomo-nosis in birds | 2-amino-5-nitro thiazole | 30 mg/kg daily for 7 days | Oral |

| | | | | |
|---|---|---|---|---|
| | | Furazolidone | 25-30 mg/kg for 7 days | Oral |
| 7. | Histomo-nosis | 2-amino-5-nitro thiazole | 0.05% preventive dose, 1% curative dose for 14 days | Oral |
| | | Dimetridazole | 0.0125% in feed | Oral |
| | | Nithiazide | 0.02% in water curative | Oral |
| | | | 0.025% in feed curative | |
| | | | 0.0125% in feed prophylactic | |
| | | Furazolidone | 0.015% as prophylactic | Oral |
| | | | 0.04% as curative | |
| 8. | Giardiosis in man | Metronidazole | 400mg tab TID 5 days – Adults. | Oral |
| | | | 5mg/kg TID for 7 days – Children | |
| | | | Second dose after 15 days | |
| | | Dimetridazole | 50mg/kg 5 days | Oral |
| | | Tinidazole | 2g single dose-Adult | Oral |
| | | | 50mg/kg - Children | |
| | | Secnidazole | 1 g tab x 2, single dose 2 g | Oral |
| 9. | Amoebiasis in man | Metronidazole | 750 mg three times a day for 5 days | Oral |
| | | Tinidazole | 2 g single dose or 50 mg/kg or 500 mg BID 5 days | Oral |
| | | Secnidazole | 2 g single dose | Oral |
| | | Ornidazole | 1.5 g single dose 500 mg BID 5-10 days | Oral |
| 10. | Chicken coccidiosis | Sulphadimidine | 0.4% in feed / 0.2% in water 3 day drug, two days rest – 3 day drug | Oral |

| | | | | |
|---|---|---|---|---|
| | | Sulphaquinoxaline | 0.43% in water 2 treatment for 2 days with 3-5 day interval | Oral |
| | | Amprolium | 0.0125% Prophylactic (Vit $B_1$, should not be given) | Oral |
| | | Nitrofurazone | 0.022% curative | Oral |
| | | Furazolidone | 0.0055% in feed | Oral |
| | | Monensin | 0.01% | Oral |
| | | Lasalocid | 0.005-0.0075% | Oral |
| | | Salinomycin | 0.01% | Oral |
| | | Maduramicin | 5-6 ppm | Oral |
| | | Toltrazuril | 75 mg/lit | Oral |
| | | Diclazuril | 1 mg/kg | Oral |
| 11. | Sheep and goat coccidiosis | Sulphaguanidine | 2 g/ day for 6 days | Oral |
| | | Nitrofurazone | 7-10 mg daily for 7 days - Feed – 0.0165% | Oral |
| | | Monensin | 22 mg/kg feed | Oral |
| | | Amprolium | 50-62.5 mg/kg for sheep<br>100 mg/kg for goat | Oral |
| | | Lasalocid | 12.5-100 mg/kg for feed | Oral |
| 12. | Bovine coccidiosis | Amprolium | 20-25 mg/kg daily feed 4-5 days | Oral |
| | | Sulphamethazine | 140 mg/kg for 3 days | Oral |
| | | Monensin | 1 mg/kg feed 10-15 days<br>16.5 g/ton feed 3-30 days | Oral |
| | | Lasalocid | 3 mg/kg in feed | Oral |
| 13. | Toxoplasmosis | Pyrimethamine | 25 mg/kg/ day 3 to 5 days - human | Oral |

| | | | | |
|---|---|---|---|---|
| | | Sulphadiazine | 4-8 g/day | I/M |
| | | Spiromycin | 2 to 4 g/day | Oral |
| 14. | Sarcocy-stosis | Sulphadiazine plus Pyrimethamine | 120 mg 1 mg/kg | I/M |
| | | 2 Suphomonyl 1-44 diamino diphenyl sulphone (SDDS) | 160-mg/kg - 3-4 days | I/M |
| | | Amprolium | 100 mg/kg - 30 days for cow | Oral |
| | | Salinomycin | 1-2 mg/kg | Oral |
| | | Halofuginone | 0.22 mg/kg | Oral |
| | | Aureomycin – Sulphamethazine premix (equal part) | 100 mg/animal | Oral |
| 15. | Avian malaria | Chloroquine | 5 mg/kg | Oral or S/C |
| | | Paludrine | 7.5 mg/kg | Oral or S/C |
| | | Pyremethamine | 0.3 mg/kg | Oral or S/C |
| | | Quinine sulphate | 0.5-1 mg | Oral |
| | | Plasmoquin | 400 mg/bird | Oral |
| 16. | Babesiosis | Diminazene aceturate | 2-3.5 mg/kg or 0.8-1.6 g/100kg | Deep I/M |
| | | Imidocarb | 0.5 to 1 mg/kg | S/C |
| | | Phenamidine 40% solution | 12 mg/kg | S/C |
| | | Pentamidine | 2-16 mg/kg | S/C or I/M |
| | | Quinacrine | 1-2mg/kg -For livestock | |
| | | | 0.25 mg/kg – For dog | S/C or I/M |
| | | Acriflavin | 20 ml of 5% aqueous solution | I/V |
| 17. | Theileriosis | Buparvaquone | 2.5 mg/kg single dose | I/M |
| | | Parvaquone | 20 mg/kg single dose | I/V |

| | | | | |
|---|---|---|---|---|
| | | Menoctone | 5-10 mg/kg curative | I/M |
| | | Halofuginone | 1-1.2 mg/kg | Oral |
| | | Chlortetracycline | 16 mg/kg for 4-7days | Oral |
| | | Tetracycline | 15 mg/kg daily for 5 days | I/V |
| 18. | Balanti-diosis | Metronidazole | 50 mg/kg for small animal<br>75 mg/kg for large animals | Oral |
| 19. | Anaplas-mosis | Long acting Oxytetracycline | 20 mg/kg | I/M |
| | | Oxytetracycline | 22 mg/kg 5 days | I/M |
| 20. | Canine ehrlichiosis | Oxytetracycline | 22 mg/kg BID for 14 days | Oral or I/V |
| | | Chlortetracycline | 22 mg/kg BID for 14 days | Oral or I/V |
| | | Doxycycline | 5 mg/kg BID for 14 days | Oral or I/V |
| | | Minocycline | 20 mg/kg BID for 14 days | Oral |
| | | Supportive therapy :<br>1. Vitamin B Complex<br>2. Liver extract<br>3. Iron dextran<br>4. Haemoglobin Tonics | | |

❑❑❑

Chapter 7

# Vaccines Against Protozoa

| S. No. | Name of the vaccine | Animal | Used against | Details |
|---|---|---|---|---|
| 1. | Leishmune | Dogs | *Leishmania donovani*- Canine visceral leishmaniasis | It contains the Fucose-Mannose-ligand (FML) antigen of *Leishmania donovani* |
| 2. | Toxovax | Sheep | *Toxoplasma gondii* | Live vaccine with $10^5$ tachyzoites of the S48 strain of *T.gondii*, a single dose 3 weeks prior to mating is given to Ewes |
| 3. | Bovilis Neoguard | Cattle | *Neospora caninum* | Killed tachyzoites Reduced abortion |
| 4. | Giardiavax | Dogs | | *Giardia duodenalis* Killed cultured trophozoites derived from sheep reduces disease as well as oocyst shedding |
| 5. | Pirodog and Nobivac piro | Dogs | *Babesia canis* | *In vitro* cultured supernatant antigen-reduces clinical disease |
| 6. | CoxAbic | Poultry | *Eimeria maxima* | 1st commercially available sub unit vaccine- Macro |

| | | | | |
|---|---|---|---|---|
| | | | | Gametocyte antigen(s) transmission blocking through maternal antibody transfer |
| 7. | Coccivac Immucox, Advent | Poultry | *Eimeria spp.* | Live Sporulated oocysts vaccine of several or all of the avian species |
| 8. | Paracox 8 | Poultry | *Eimeria spp.* | Live attenuated oral vaccine having oocysts derived from 8 precocious lines of coccidia |
| 9. | Nobilis Cox ATM | Poultry | *Eimeria spp.* | It has a special property of being active in the presence of ionophore compounds. Contains *E.acervulina, E.tenella and E.maxima* |
| 10. | Inovocox | Poultry | *Eimeria spp.* | In ovo delivery using proprietary platform injection system |
| 11. | Livacox | Poultry | *Eimeria tenella* | Precocious and egg passaged lines |
| 12. | Rakshavac T | Cattle | *Theileria annulata* | Schizont infected lymphoblast cell culture vaccine |
| 13. | Epm vaccine | Horses | *Sarcocystis neurona* | *In vitro* cultured merozoites, chemically inactivated |
| 14. | Trichguard | Cattle | *Tritrichomonas foetus* | Killed vaccine |
| 15. | Anaplaz Anavac Plazvax | Cattle | *Anaplasma* | Killed vaccine Modified live vaccine Inactivated vaccine |

□□□

Chapter 8

# Fill Up the Blanks

1. Trypanosomes have ............................... type of nucleus
2. Thut in elephants is caused by ...............................
3. LD bodies are nothing but the ................................ stage of *Leishmania donovani*
4. Promastigotes of *Leishmania* are seen in ............................... and ...............................
5. Sabin Feldman dye test is used in the diagnosis of ................... ...........................
6. Flagella is the organelle used for ...............................
7. Flagella arises from ............................... in the cytoplasm
8. Abortion during the 1st trimester of pregnancy in cattle is caused by ............................... protozoan.
9. Chancre is the 1st visible lesion seen in ...............................
10. Romana's sign is pathognomonic of ........................................ infection
11. Chronic infection with ............................... protozoan results in mega colon condition in man
12. The only trypanosome transmitted by the venereal route is ...............................

13. Corneal opacity and laryngeal oedema in dogs is due to .............................. protozoan infection

14. Extreme emaciation, with bag of bone like condition in horses is associated with .............................. infection

15. Sulphur yellow coloured dropping in turkeys is indicative of .............................. infection

16. The caecal worm of poultry, *Heterakis gallinae* is instrumental in the transmission of .............................. protozoans to turkeys

17. Cervical lymphadenopathy in man associated with *Trypanosoma gambiense* is also referred to as..............................

18. The first parasitic protozoa discovered was ..............................

19. The macronuclei of ciliates is associated with .............................. function

20. Osmoregulatory organelles in protozoa are ..............................

21. Single cell in which the nucleus is undergoing several divisions is termed ..............................

22. Trypanosomes which develop in the vector in the posterior part of the alimentary tract belong to the section ..............................

23. Characteristic flask shaped ulcers in the large intestine in man is associated with .............................. protozoa

24. Plastic granules in the macrogamont is associated with the function of .............................. formation in the oocyst

25. Eimerian oocyst has .............................. number of sporocysts with .............................. sporozoites while Isosporan oocyst has .............................. number of sporocysts with .............................. sporozoites

26. Caecal coccidiosis in chicken is caused by ..............................

27. Pigeon malaria is caused by ..............................

28. Malarial parasites present in the erythrocytes begin to multiply to produce disease. This type of relapse is called ..............................

29. The schizonts of *Theileria annulata* are commonly referred to as .............................. and they are present in the .............................. cells

30. ................................ stages in the life cycle of *Theileria annulata* have been attenuated to produce the vaccine Rakshavac T

31. The drug of choice for *Theileria annulata* is ................................

32. ................................ drug is used in the prophylactic and therapeutic treatment of trypanosomosis

33. Pelta is a structure associated with ................................ protozoan

34. ................................ is a tissue invading coccidian which is congenitally transmitted in both dogs and cattle.

35. Horses can be protected against *Trypanosoma evansi* infection by giving a dose of ................................ drug.

36. Immunologic intradermal test to detect *Leishmania tropica* is ................................

37. Sporulation of oocysts requires ................................ and ................................ environmental conditions

38. The only stage in the life cycle of coccidian possessing flagella is the ................................

39. Vector of *Leishmania tropica* is ................................

40. Chromatoid bodies are seen in ................................ protozoa

41. The micronuclei of ciliates is responsible for the ................................ function of the organism

42. ................................ is the false feet of *Entamoeba histolytica* used for locomotion

43. ................................ is a process by which many protozoa ingest nutrient material by pinching off of vacuoles of fluid through temporary opening in the body wall.

44. The process of multiple fission of the zygote is termed ................................ and the uninucleate cells produced are the ................................

45. Dum dum fever is caused by ................................

46. Xenodiagnosis has been used in the diagnosis of ................................

47. The first protozoa was discovered by ................................

48. The vegetative motile form of the protozoa is termed ..............................

49. An example of a stercorarian trypanosome is ..............................

50. The only trypanosome which invades cells is ..............................

51. Salivarian trypanosomes are transmitted through the .............................. of vector while the stercorarian trypanosomes are transmitted through .............................. contamination

52. The only pathogenic stercorarian trypanosome affecting man is ..............................

53. Dollar spot lesions are characteristic of .............................. disease

54. The amastigote stage of *Leishmania* is also known as ..............................

55. Blood smears are fixed with ..............................

56. Terminal kinetoplast is seen in ..............................

57. PKADL is a complication of ..............................

58. Canker or Yellow button lesions or Yellow caseous nodules in the crop of pigeons is caused by ..............................

59. *Trichomonas gallinae* infection is transmitted from adult pigeons to pigeon squabs through ..............................

60. Salt and pepper markings in the mid intestine of chicken is caused by ..............................

61. .............................. is the infective stage in chicken coccidiosis

62. Black head or Cyanotic head in turkeys is the pathognomonic lesion in infection with ..............................

63. Raptors and predatory birds preying upon pigeons are likely to get infection with ..............................

64. The trypanosome commonly called as Occult, Cryptic or Hidden trypanosome is ..............................

65. Metrocytes are seen inside ..............................

66. .............................. is called cell eating and .............................. is called cell drinking

67. ................................ act as both intermediate and definitive host for *Toxoplasma gondii.*

68. Two types of oocyst, one with thin wall and another with thick wall is produced by ................................

69. Phanerozoites and Cryptozoites are associated with the life cycle of ................................ protozoan

70. Globoid or giant schizonts are characteristic of ................................ coccidian of cattle.

71. Only mature ................................ nucleated *Entamoeba histolytica* are infective to man.

72. Punched out ulcers in abomasums and infarcts in kidney are characteristic lesions in cattle caused by ................................

73. Megaoesophagus and Megacolon in human beings are features of ................................ disease

74. Haemoglobinuria/brown or red coloured urine/coffee coloured urine in cattle is a striking feature of ................................

75. The protozoan infection characterized by prescapular lymph node swelling, high fever and grinding of teeth in cattle is ................................

76. Loss of hump in camels is seen in infection with ......................

77. Yellowish green necrotic lesions in liver of turkeys is caused by ................................

78. Babies will be born dead or alive with extreme symptoms like hydrocephalus, retino-choroiditis, cerebral calcification and encephalitis referred to as " tetrad of signs" are affected with ................................

79. Bean shaped macronucleus is seen in ................................

80. Oocyst with four naked sporozoites is a feature of ..........................

81. Dumb bell shaped oocyst is found in ................................

82. Maltese cross formation in RBC of horses is characteristic of ................................

83. Halter shaped gamont (halteridium) in pigeon RBC belongs to ................................

84. Rakshavac T is a vaccine against ..............................

85. Actively multiplying forms in the life cycle of *Toxoplasma gondii* are .............................. whereas slow multiplying forms are ..............................

86. Inverse age resistance is a feature of .............................. in calves

87. Premunity is a feature of ..............................

88. Early abortion in the first trimester of pregnancy in cattle is caused by the protozoa ..............................

89. Raineys corpuscles are associated with ..............................

90. Sir Ronald Ross was awarded Nobel prize for his pioneering work on the discovery of the causative agent for ................ ..............

91. Conjugation is a mode of reproduction in ..............................

92. Movement in *Toxoplasma gondii* is by ..............................

93. A trypanosome that does not require a vector is ..........................

94. Endogenous sporulation of oocysts occurs in ..............................

95. In thick blood smear preparation at first the slide is dipped in water for few minutes to get rid of the haemoglobin. This process is called .............................. or ..............................

96. Malabsorption and steatorrhea in man is caused by ................ .............

97. *Toxoplasma gondii* multiplies by ..............................

98. Ladder like lesions in the intestine of chicken is caused by ..............................

99. Polyp like lesion in the intestine of goat is produced by ................ ..............

100. Locomotion in *Balantidium coli* is by ..............................

101. Motile zygote of *Plasmodium gallinaceum* is called as ....................

102. Shuttle programme/Rotation programe is one of the medication program for control of ..............................

103. Relapse or Recrudescence is a feature of ..............................

104. Protozoan disease which is self limiting in cows is ..........................

105. Transmission of protozoan diseases by ticks through eggs is called ................................ and through various tick stages is called ................................

106. ................................ is a classic example of obligatory and facultative heteroxenus life cycle

107. British Veterinarian in India who was behind the discovery of *Trypanosoma evansi* is ................................

108. Miescher's tubules are associated with ................................

109. Apical complex is a structure in ................................

110. Iodine staining is used to detect the cysts of ................................

111. ................................ stage is the most pathogenic in the life cycle of *Eimeria tenella* and causes the maximum damage

112. ................................ type of nucleus found in ciliates

113. ................................ fly plays a major role in transmission of *Entamoeba histolytica*

114. The first generation pre-erythrocytic schizonts of *Plasmodium gallinaceum* is termed as ................................

115. Monkey face or Smiley face mimicking protozoa is ..........................

116. Examination of cerebrospinal fluid is one of the important diagnostic methods for ..............................

117. Trypanosomes are grouped into ................................ and ................................ depending on the site of development in vector

118. Various parts of the cell of protozoa performing various activities is called ..............................

119. ................................ and ................................ are the two types of nucleus in protozoa

120. Two types of compact nuclei in ciliates are ................................ and ................................

121. ................................ are whip like organelles used for locomotion in trypanosomes

122. .................................. are eye lash like organelles used for locomotion in *Balantidium coli*

123. Cytoplasm in protozoa is divided into an outer dense hyaline portion ........................ and inner granular portion ......................

124. In .............................. nutrition protozoa synthesize food from inorganic materials

125. Temporary mouth in some protozoa is called ............................... and temporary excretory opening is called ...............................

126. ............................... and .............................. are the two types of binary fission in protozoa

127. Longitudinal binary fission occurs in ................................ and transverse binary fission occurs in ...............................

128. In Schizogony, the dividing cell is called ............................... and the daughter cells are known as ...............................

129. In *Toxoplasma gondii*, many daughter cells are produced from a parent cell by a process of ..............................

130. Internal budding in which two daughter cells are formed from the mother cell is called ..............................

131. Internal budding producing more than two daughter cells is ............................... whereas external budding more than two daughter cells is ..............................

132. The two types of sexual reproduction in protozoa are ................... ........... and ..............................

133. In .............................. two individual protozoa come together temporarily, fuse together and exchange of genetic material occurs

134. .............................. is the process of union of male and female gametes to form zygote

135. Gametes of similar size are called ............................... and gametes with dissimilar size are called ..............................

136. The smaller male gamete is called ............................... and larger female gamete is called ..............................

137. The process of gamete formation is called ...............................

138. The process of fusion of two identical gametes is called ............................... and fusion of two dissimilar gametes is called ...............................

139. The process by which zygote is divided to form a number of sporozoites is called ...............................

140. ............................... have leaf like body, flagella and undulating membrane

141. Surra means ...............................

142. *Trypanosoma evansi* transmitted by *Tabanus sp.* is an example of ............................... transmission whereas African trypanosomes transmitted by *Glossina sp.* is an example of ............................... transmission

143. In the life cycle of trypanosomes infection is transmitted by inoculation by arthropod vectors in ............................... development and infection occurs by contamination of skin or skin wound in ............................... development

144. In ............................... stage of trypanosomes kinetoplast and flagella are at anterior tip of body with no undulating membrane

145. ............................... stage of trypanosomes flagella is just anterior to nucleus and undulating membrane is short

146. ............................... stage of trypanosome is seen normally in blood of infected animals

147. Haemolytic anemia, hypoglycemia, erythrophagocytosis and disseminating intravascular coagulation are pathological conditions caused by ...............................

148. ............................... , ............................... , ............................... and ............................... are non specific chemical tests to diagnose trypanosomosis

149. ............................... protein is responsible for antigenic variation in trypanosomes and hence no vaccine could be developed

150. ............................... is the largest trypanosome

151. NNN media used for culture of trypanosomes is ...............................

152. Nagana is derived from a Zulu term which means ...............................

153. Wild animals like opossums, raccoons and armadillos are reservoirs for ................................

154. ................................ and ................................ are the two drugs available for treatment of Chagas Disease

155. Protozoa of cattle transmitted by coitus, improper Artificial insemination equipments and use of contaminated speculum is ................................

156. Site of predilection of *Tritrichomonas foetus* in bull is ................................ and cow is ................................

157. Early abortion at 1-16 weeks after successful breeding in cows is characteristic of infection with protozoa ................................

158. The four forms of *Histomonas meleagridis* are ................................, ................................, ................................ and ................................

159. Characteristic depressed saucer shaped circular yellow to yellowish green areas of necrosis in liver of turkeys is caused by ................................

160. Cyanotic comb and wattle in turkeys is caused by infection with ................................

161. Separate rearing of chicken and turkeys is an important management practice to prevent infection with ................................

162. Enzyme that assist in the pathogenesis of *Entamoeba histolytica* and *Balantidium coli* in spreading the lesions is ................................

163. Commonest location of amoebic abscess in liver in human beings is the ................................ lobe

164. Micropyle, polar cap, stieda body and contractile vacuole are structures seen in the ................................ of *Eimeria sp.*

165. Drugs that are used to kill coccidia are called ................................ and drugs that are used to control the multiplication of coccidia are called ................................

166. The most pathogenic coccidia affecting cattle is ................................

167. In cattle, infection with ................................ causes severe tenesmus, bloody diarrhea, emaciation, dehydration and sunken eyes and hind quarter of affected animals looks like as if they are smeared with red paint

168. In *Eimeria bovis* schizogony occurs in ............................... and gametogony occurs in ...............................

169. Mature schizont of ............................... is visible to naked eye as whitish balls (400 μm) and is useful in identification

170. Two generation of schizogony with giant first generation schizonts called megaloschizonts are observed in ...............................

171. Zoonotically important cyst forming protozoa discovered by Nicolle and Manceaux is ...............................

172. Tachyzoite of *Toxoplasma gondii* is ............................... shaped

173. Three infective stages of *Toxoplasma gondii* are ..........................., ............................... and ...............................

174. In *Toxoplasma gondii,* tachyzoites multiply by repeated endodyogeny within the host cell till it is filled with crescent shaped zoites enclosed in a parasitophorous vacuole and this structure is termed as ...............................

175. Bradyzoites of *Toxoplasma gondii* are ............................... in shape

176. Two developmental cycles in the transmission of *Toxoplasma gondii* are ............................... and ...............................

177. In sheep, abortion storms, neonatal mortality, mummification of foetus and birth of weak lambs is caused by ...............................

178. Two types of Toxoplasmosis in human beings are .............................. and ...............................

179. Tachyzoites of *Sarcocystis cruzi* are also termed as .......................

180. Protrusions seen in the Sarcocyst wall are called as ..................

181. Immature sarcocyst contains globular merozoites called ....................................... which then undergo endodyogeny leading to crescent/banana/sickle shaped zoites called ...............................

182. The RBC pigment formed from host haemoglobin in Malaria is ...............................

183. In *Plasmodium gallinaceum* infection, schizogony occurs in .......................... and sexual phase occurs in ............................

184. Cryptozoites, Metacryptozoites and Phanerozoites are seen in the life cycle of ..............................

185. Gelatin capsule shaped gamonts inside neutrophils of dogs belong to ..............................

186. Protozoa of dogs which is acquired by ingestion of infected brown dog tick is ..............................

187. Two types of meronts, macromeronts and micromeronts are seen in the life cycle of ..............................

188. Babesiosis caused by *Babesia bigemina* in cattle is transmitted by .............................. through *Boophilus ( Rhipicephalus ) microplus* ticks whereas *Babesia canis* in dogs is transmitted by .............................. through *Rhipicephalus sanguineus* ticks

189. .............................. sp. of protozoa are found in pairs in RBC and are pear shaped

190. Ray bodies or Strahlenkorper's bodies are seen in the life cycle of ..............................

191. Merozoites or piroplasms of *Theileria annulata* are found inside .............................. and schizonts are found inside ..............................

192. In the life cycle of *Theileria annulata* ovoid or spherical zygotes are transformed to club shaped mobile structures called ..............................

193. A most important protozoan disease causing lymphoproliferation in cattle is ..............................

194. The ciliate protozoa found in colon of pigs and primates and is a problem in zoological gardens is ..............................

195. .............................. is the ciliate protozoa which is actively motile and moves quickly over the microscopic field

196. Macronucleus of *Balantidium coli* is .............................. or .............................. shaped

197. *Balantidium coli* reproduces by .............................. and ..............................

198. In birds, infection with .............................. is characterized by hemoptysis and severe renal lesion

199. ................................ mosquitoes are vectors for human malaria and .............................. mosquitoes are vectors for bird malaria

200. The word malaria means ..............................

201. The mature schizont of *Plasmodium gallinaceum* is called ..............................

202. Morula or Mulberry forms typical of *Ehrlichia sp* are found inside ..............................

203. Epistaxis, pancytopenia, thrombocytopenia and petechiae of skin in dogs is caused by ..............................

204. Rakshavac T vaccine is a .............................. culture vaccine used for prevention of theileriosis

205. Spinner flash suspension culture and microaerophilic stationary phase culture technique is used to cultivate ..............................

206. Theileriosis is transmitted by ..............................

207. The *Babesia sp.* in which exoerythrocytic schizogony occurs with development of macro and micro schizont in lymphoblastoid cell *in vitro* and *in vivo* is ..............................

208. In the life cycle of *Babesia sp,* the cytomere is differentiated which release vermiform shaped several kinetes called .................... ........... or ..............................

209. The *Babesia sp.* which causes multiple infection of erythrocytes in which sometimes more than 16 organisms can be found in a single RBC is ..............................

210. CNS damage in case of infection with *Babesia bovis* and *Babesia canis* occurs due to ..............................

211. Trypanosome surface coat has .............................. enzyme which break down sialic acid in the RBC surface causing erythrolysis

212. Anemia in trypanosomosis is ..............................

213. The powerful endotoxin produced by *Sarcocystis sp.* is ..............................

214. Hypnozoites are associated with the life cycle of ......................

215. Villus atrophy with flat mucosa syndrome in goats is caused by ..............................

216. The vitamin which is contraindicated in chicken administered with amprolium for control of coccidiosis is ...............................

217. In chicken, infection with ............................... intestinal contents consist of pinkish mucoid exudates or orange slimy exudates

218. Balooning of caeca and intestine with blood filled contents are characteristic of infection with ............................... and ............................... , respectively

219. Bloody droppings in chicken is the first sign in infection with ...............................

220. The most pathogenic *Eimeria* sp of chicken is ...............................

221. *Eimeria* sp of chicken which interfere with the absorption of xanthophyll and carotenoid pigment is ...............................

222. In *Eimeria maxima* more serious pathogenic effects are caused due to ...............................

223. The three factors responsible for excystment of coccidian oocyst are ........................... , ........................... and ...........................

224. The structure found in sporozoite/merozoite of coccidian used for penetration of host cell is ...............................

225. Vitamins that has to be given as supplementation in coccidiosis infected chicken is ............................... and ...............................

226. Hepatic coccidiosis in rabbits is caused by ...............................

227. Renal coccidiosis in goose is caused by ...............................

□□□

Chapter 9

# Multiple Choice Questions

1. Development stage of trypanosome with rounded body with a degenerated fibril of flagellum is the

   A. Trypomastigote stage B. Amastigote stage

   C. Promastigote stage D. Epimastigote stage

2. *Tritrichomonas foetus* move using

   A. Subpellicular microtubules

   B. Cilia

   C. Flagella

   D. Pseudopodia

3. The following trypanosome belongs to section Stercoraria

   A. *Trypanosoma evansi* B. *Trypanosoma equiperdum*

   C. *Trypanosoma theileri* D. *Trypanosoma brucei*

4. Xenodiagnosis is commonly used to diagnose

   A. *Trypanosoma evansi* B. *Trypanosoma equiperdum*

   C. *Trypanosoma theileri* D. *Trypanosoma cruzi*

5. The media used to culture *Trichomonas* is

A. NNN media
B. Diamonds media
C. Ringer's media
D. Balamuth's media

6. The only coccidian with two morphofunctional occysts is

A. *Eimeria maxima*
B. *Cryptosporidium parvum*
C. *Toxoplasma gondii*
D. *Isospora felis*

7. The coccidia of poultry with low pathogenicity and maximum immunizing capacity is

A. *Eimeria tenella*
B. *Eimeria necatrix*
C. *Eimeria maxima*
D. *Eimeria brunetti*

8. Plasma Kallikrein play an important role in the pathogenesis of

A. *Babesia bigemina*
B. *Theileria annulata*
C. *Babesia bovis*
D. *Trypanosoma evansi*

9. Schaudinns haemotoxylin staining method is used to diagnose

A. *Cryptosporidium*
B. *Entamoeba histolytica*
C. *Eimeria bovis*
D. *Toxoplasma gondii*

10. Sporocysts are absent in

A. *Cryptosporidium*
B. *Neospora caninum*
C. *Eimeria bovis*
D. *Toxoplasma gondii*

11. The first report of tropical bovine theileriosis in India was made by

A. Ronald Ross
B. Chandler
C. Alfred Lingard
D. Leishman and Donovan

12. *Theileria mutans* in cattle is a

A. Lymphoproliferative type
B. Hemoproliferative type
C. Tissue proliferative type
D. None of the above

13. Romana's sign is pathognomonic for infection with

A. *Trypanosoma gambiense* B. *Trypanosoma cruzi*

C. *Trypanosoma rhodesiense* D. *Trypanosoma evansi*

14. The most pathogenic stage in the life cycle of *Theileria annulata* is

A. Merozoite B. Schizont

C. Trophozoite D. Gamont

15. The prepatent period of *Toxoplasma gondii* is shortest when a cat ingests

A. Oocysts B. Tachyzoites

C. Bradyzoites D. Sporozoites

16. Coccidian oocysts can be sporulated in the laboratory by placing the dung in

A. 2.5% potassium dichromate

B. 10% Sodium hydroxide

C. 10% Potassium hydroxide

D. 1% alcohol

17. Lymphadenopathy resulting in winterbottom sign in man is due to

A. *Trypanosoma brucei* B. *Trypanosoma gambiense*

C. *Trypanosoma rhodesiense* D. *Trypanosoma cruzi*

18. Xenodiagnosis is commonly employed to detect

A. *Leishmania donovani* B. *Trypanosoma cruzi*

C. *Trypanosoma theileri* D. *Leishmania tropica*

19. Atovaquone and Azithromycin is used in the treatment of

A. *Babesia canis* B. *Babesia gibsoni*

C. *Trypanosoma evansi* D. *Hepatozoon canis*

20. Immune evasion by antgenic variation is a common phenomenon in

A. *Babesia canis* B. *Babesia gibsoni*

C. *Trypanosoma evansi* D. *Hepatozoon canis*

21. Rectal coccidiosis in birds is caused by

A. *Eimeria necatrix* B. *Eimeria maxima*

C. *Eimeria tenella* D. *Eimeria brunetti*

22. Cerebral babesiosis is caused by

A. *Babesia bovis* B. *Babesia bigemina*

C. *Babesia gibsoni* D. *Babesia ovis*

23. N dama cattle represents animals which are resistant to

A. *Babesia bigemina* B. *Theileria annulata*

C. *Babesia bovis* D. *Trypanosoma evansi*

24. Rigid paralysis with hyperextension of hind limbs in dogs is due to

A. *Babesia canis* B. *Neospora caninum*

C. *Trypanosoma evansi* D. *Hepatozoon canis*

25. Nutrition in which organism utilizes preformed food from living animals or plants is

A. Holophytic B. Autotrophic

C. Holozoic D. Saprozoic

26. When protozoa forms a heavy wall around itself it is called

A. Cyst B. Pseudocyst

C. Spore D. Trophozoite

27. Fatal termination is more likely in the case of human trypanosomosis caused by

A. *Trypanosoma brucei* B. *Trypanosoma gambiense*

C. *Trypanosoma rhodesiense* D. *Trypanosoma cruzi*

28. The largest trypanosome affecting livestock and humans is

A. *Trypanosoma brucei* B. *Trypanosoma evansi*

C. *Trypanosoma rhodesiense* D. *Trypanosoma theileri*

29. The crescent shaped schizotrypanum affecting man is

A. *Trypanosoma brucei* B. *Trypanosoma gambiense*

C. *Trypanosoma rhodesiense* D. *Trypanosoma cruzi*

30. The smallest African trypanosome is

A. *Trypanosoma brucei* B. *Trypanosoma congolense*

C. *Trypanosoma vivax* D. *Trypanosoma cruzi*

31. In *Trypanosoma congolense* the kinetoplast is medium sized and placed

A. Subterminal

B. Terminal

C. Marginal

D. Between the nucleus and the posterior blunt end

32. *Trypanosoma cruzi* is seen within the tissue cells in the ________ ____________ stage

A. Amastigote B. Trypomastigote

C. Promastigote D. Epimastigote

33. Dalmeny disease in cows is considered to be associated with the protozoan

A. *Toxoplasma gondii* B. *Sarcocystis cruzi*

C. *Trypanosoma theileri* D. *Neospora caninum*

34. The first report of the an arthropod transmitting a protozoan was made by

A. Ronald Ross B. Smith and Kilbourne

C. Alfred Lingard D. Leishman and Donovan

35. *Tritrichomonas foetus* multiplies by

A. Conjugation B. Schizogony

C. Transverse binary fission D. Longitudinal binary fission

36. Pick the odd pair of protozoan disease and drug of choice

A. Theileriosis - Buparvaquone

B. Sarcocystosis - Furazolidone

C. Amoebic dysentery - Tinidazole

D. Babesiosis – Diminazine aceturate

37. J.P. Dubey is a renowned scientist associated with

A. Theileriosis B. Toxoplasmosis

C. Trypanosomosis D. Tritrichomonosis

38. The first subunit vaccine against poultry coccidiosis Cox Abic contains

A. Schizonts B. Merozoites

C. Trophozoite D. Gametocyte

39. Toxovax, a vaccine against Toxoplasmosis prevents

A. Schizogony B. Oocyst formation

C. Trophozoite penetration D. Sporozoite activation

40. Pick out the protozoa not seen in blood

A. *Toxoplasma* B. *Sarcocystis*

C. *Cryptosporidium* D. *Theileria*

❏❏❏

Chapter 10

# Frequently Asked Subjective Questions

## Short Notes

1. Locomotion in protozoa
2. Reproduction in protozoa
3. Difference between salivarian and stercorarian trypanosomes
4. Developmental stages of trypanosomes
5. Dourine
6. PKADL
7. Pigeon canker
8. Factors which influence the outbreak of coccidiosis in poultry
9. Winter coccidiosis in cattle
10. Depict the structure of a sporulated oocyst
11. How will you differentiate between an isosporan and Eimerian oocyst
12. Cryptosporidiosis
13. Abortion storm in sheep
14. *Neospora caninum*
15. Structure of Sarcocyst

16. Pigeon malaria
17. Kochs blue bodies
18. Advantages and disadvantages of thick and thin blood smears
19. Cerebral babesiosis
20. Travelers' diarhoea
21. Role of *Heterakis gallinarum* in transmission of *Histomonas meleagridis*
22. Chronic chagas disease
23. Cutaneous leishmaniasis
24. Sleeping sickness in man
25. Xenodiagnosis
26. Phanerozoites
27. Avian malaria
28. *Balantidium coli*
29. Rakshavac T
30. Sporulation of coccidia in the laboratory
31. Giemsa staining technique
32. Wet film examination
33. Microhaematocrit method in the detection of protozoans
34. Cryptic trypanosome
35. Diagram of *Tritrichomonas foetus*
36. Diagnosis of *Trypanosoma evansi*
37. Difference between Eukaryotes and prokaryotes
38. Vaccines against poultry coccidia
39. Types of protozoan nucleus
40. OPG

## Essay

1. Give an account of surra in animals
2. Write the mode of transmission, pathogenesis, clinical signs and control of *Tritrichomonas foetus*
3. List the coccidian affecting poultry and give a detailed account of caecal coccidiosis
4. Diagrammatically represent the life cycle of *Eimeria necatrix*. Write the pathogenesis, treatment and control of intestinal coccidiosis
5. Give a detailed account of toxoplasmosis in man and animals
6. Red water fever in cattle
7. Write in detail about tropical bovine theileriosis
8. An cross bred calf is presented in the large animal ward with history of fever, being off feed and sudden reduction in milk yield. Palpation of the prescalpular lymph node reveals lymphadenitis. Lymph node biopsy reveals the presence of schizonts in the the lymphocytes. What is your diagnosis. How will you proceed with the treatment and control of this infection
9. Give an account of the vaccines produced against protozoans in India and abroad
10. Depict the life cycle of *Babesia bigemina* and discuss the pathogenic effect of the protozoan
11. Give a detailed account of the life cycle, pathogenesis, treatment and control of *Entamoeba histolytica*
12. Write in detail about the tissue invading coccidia
13. List the Romanovsky's stains. Compare and contrast between Giemsa and Leishman staining techniques
14. Discuss the methods involved in taking a blood smear, the types of blood smears, advantages and disadvantages and examination of blood smears

□□□

Chapter 11

# Important Text Books in Veterinary Protozoology


1. Helminths, Arthropods and Protozoa of domesticated animals - E.J.L. Soulsby
2. Veterinary Protozoology - Norman D. Levine
3. Veterinary Parasitology - G.M. Urquhart, J. Armour, J.L. Duncan, A.M. Dunn and F.W. Jennings
4. Textbook of Veterinary Protozoology - B.B. Bhatia
5. Veterinary Parasitology - M.A. Taylor, R.L. Koop and R.L. Wall

Chapter 12

# Answers - Fill Up the Blanks

1. Vesicular
2. *Trypanosoma evansi*
3. Amastigote
4. Vector, cultures
5. Toxoplasmosis
6. Locomotion
7. Kinetosome or blepharoplast
8. *Tritrichomonas foetus*
9. African trypanosomosis
10. *Trypanosoma cruzi*
11. *Trypanosoma cruzi*
12. *Trypanosoma equiperdum*
13. *Trypanosoma evansi*
14. *Trypanosoma evansi*
15. *Histomonas meleagridis*
16. *Histomonas meleagridis*
17. Winterbottom's sign

18. *Eimeria stiedae*
19. Vegetative
20. Contractile vacuoles
21. Schizont/meront/segmenter/gamont
22. Stercorarian
23. *Entamoeba histolytica*
24. Wall
25. Four, two, two, four
26. *Eimeria tenella*
27. *Haemoproteus columbae*
28. Recrudescence
29. Koch's blue bodies, lymphocyte
30. Schizont
31. Buparvaquone
32. Antrycide prosalt
33. *Trichomonas gallinae*
34. *Neospora caninum*
35. Antrycide prosalt
36. Montenegro test or intradermal leishmanin test
37. Moisture, temperature
38. Microgamete
39. *Phlebotomus sergenti*
40. *Entamoeba histolytica*
41. Reproduction
42. Pseudopodia
43. Pinocytosis
44. Sporogony, sporozoites
45. *Leishmania donovani*

46. *Trypanosoma cruzi*
47. Antonie van Leeuwenhoek
48. Trophozoite
49. *Trypanosoma cruzi/Trypanosoma theileri/Trypanosoma melophagium*
50. *Trypanosoma cruzi*
51. Bite, faecal
52. *Trypanosoma cruzi*
53. Dourine
54. Leishman Donovan bodies or LD bodies
55. Methanol
56. *Trypanosoma vivax*
57. Visceral leishmaniosis
58. *Trichomonas gallinae*
59. Crop milk
60. *Eimeria necatrix*
61. Sporulated oocyst
62. *Histomonas meleagridis*
63. *Trichomonas gallinae*
64. *Trypanosoma theileri*
65. Sarcocyst
66. Phagocytosis, Pinocytosis
67. Cat
68. *Cryptosporidium parvum*
69. *Plasmodium*
70. *Eimeria bovis*
71. Four nuclei or quadrinucleate
72. *Theileria annulata*
73. Chagas disease

74. Babesiosis
75. Theileriosis
76. *Trypanosoma evansi*
77. *Histomonas meleagridis*
78. *Toxoplasma gondii*
79. *Balantidium coli*
80. *Cryptosporidium parvum*
81. *Sarcocystis cruzi*
82. *Theileria equi*
83. *Haemoproteus columbae*
84. *Theileria annulata*
85. Tachyzoites, bradyzoites
86. Babesiosis
87. Theileriosis
88. *Tritrichomonas foetus*
89. *Sarcocystis cruzi*
90. Bird malaria
91. *Balantidium coli*
92. Gliding
93. *Trypanosoma equiperdum*
94. *Sarcocystis cruzi*
95. Laking or dehaemoglobinization
96. *Giardia lamblia*
97. Endodyogeny
98. *Eimeria acervulina*
99. *Eimeria arloingi*
100. Cilia
101. Ookinete

102. Coccidiosis in chicken
103. Avian malaria
104. Trichomonosis
105. Transovarian transmission, trans stadial transmission
106. *Toxoplasma gondii*
107. Griffith Evans
108. Sarcocyst
109. *Eimeria sp.*
110. *Entamoeba histolytica*
111. Second generation schizonts
112. Compact
113. House fly
114. Cryptozoites
115. *Giardia lamblia*
116. *Toxoplasma gondii*
117. Salivarian, stercorarian
118. Organelle
119. Vesicular, compact
120. Micronucleus, macronucleus
121. Flagella
122. Cilia
123. Ectoplasm, endoplasm
124. Autotrophic
125. Cytostome, cytopyge or cell anus
126. Longitudinal, transverse
127. Flagellates, ciliates
128. Meront / schizont / segmentor / agamont, merozoites or schizozoites

129. Budding
130. Endodyogeny
131. Endopolygeny, ectopolygeny
132. Conjugation, syngamy
133. Conjugation
134. Syngamy
135. Isogametes, anisogametes
136. Microgamete, macrogamete
137. Gametogony or gamogony
138. Isogamy, anisogamy or heterogamy
139. Sporogony
140. Trypanosomes
141. Rotten or putrified
142. Mechanical, cyclical
143. Anterior station or salivarian, posterior station or stercorarian
144. Promastigote
145. Epimastigote
146. Trypomastigote
147. *Trypanosoma evansi*
148. Stilbamidine test, mercuric chloride test, formal gel test, nitric acid test
149. Variable surface glycoprotein or VSG
150. *Trypanosoma theileri* or *Trypanosoma himalayanum*
151. Novy McNeal Nicolle
152. To be in low or depressed spirits
153. *Trypanosoma cruzi*
154. Benznidazole, nifurtimox
155. *Tritrichomonas foetus*

156. Preputial cavity, genital tract
157. *Tritrichomonas foetus*
158. Invasive, vegetative, resistant, flagellar
159. *Histomonas meleagridis*
160. *Histomonas meleagridis*
161. *Histomonas meleagridis*
162. Hyaluronidase
163. Right
164. Oocyst
165. Coccidiocidal, coccidiostat
166. *Eimeria zuernii*
167. *Eimeria zuernii*
168. Small intestine, caecum, colon and terminal ileum
169. *Eimeria bovis*
170. *Eimeria arloingi*
171. *Toxoplasma gondii*
172. Arc/crescent/comma
173. Tachyzoites, bradyzoites, sporozoites
174. Clone or pseudocyst
175. Spherical
176. Enteroepithelial cycle, extraintestinal cycle
177. *Toxoplasma gondii*
178. Congenitally acquired, post natally acquired
179. Rainey's corpuscles
180. Cytophaneres
181. Metrocytes or mother cells, bradyzoites
182. Haemozoin
183. Endothelial cells of definitive host, mosquitoes

184. *Plasmodium gallinaceum*
185. *Hepatozoon canis*
186. *Hepatozoon canis*
187. *Hepatozoon canis*
188. Transovarian transmission, trans stadial transmission
189. *Babesia*
190. *Babesia bigemina*
191. RBC, lymphocyte
192. Kinetes
193. *Theileria*
194. *Balantidium coli*
195. *Balantidium coli*
196. Kidney, sausage
197. Transverse binary fission, conjugation
198. *Leucocytozoon caulleryi*
199. Anopheline, Culicine
200. Bad air
201. Segmenter
202. Monocytes
203. *Ehrlichia canis*
204. Schizont infected lymphoblast
205. *Babesia*
206. Trans stadially
207. *Babesia equi*
208. Sporokinete, vermicules
209. *Babesia canis*
210. Blockage of brain capillaries by parasitized cells
211. Sialase

212. Normocytic normochromic
213. Sarcocystin
214. *Isospora felis*
215. *Eimeria arloingi*
216. Vitamin B1 (Thiamine)
217. *Eimeria maxima*
218. *Eimeria tenella, Eimeria necatrix*
219. Coccidiosis
220. *Eimeria tenella*
221. *Eimeria maxima*
222. Sexual stage (gamonts)
223. $CO_2$, trypsin, bile
224. Apical complex
225. Vit K, Vit A
226. *Eimeria stiedae*
227. *Eimeria truncata*

## Multiple choice questions

1. B
2. C
3. C
4. D
5. B
6. B
7. C
8. A
9. B
10. A
11. C
12. B
13. B
14. B
15. C
16. A
17. B
18. B
19. B
20. C

| | |
|---|---|
| 21. D | 22. A |
| 23. D | 24. B |
| 25. D | 26. C |
| 27. D | 28. A |
| 29. D | 30. B |
| 31. A | 32. A |
| 33. B | 34. B |
| 35. D | 36. B |
| 37. B | 38. D |
| 39. B | 40. C |

□□□

# Annexures

## Annexure I: Helminth eggs

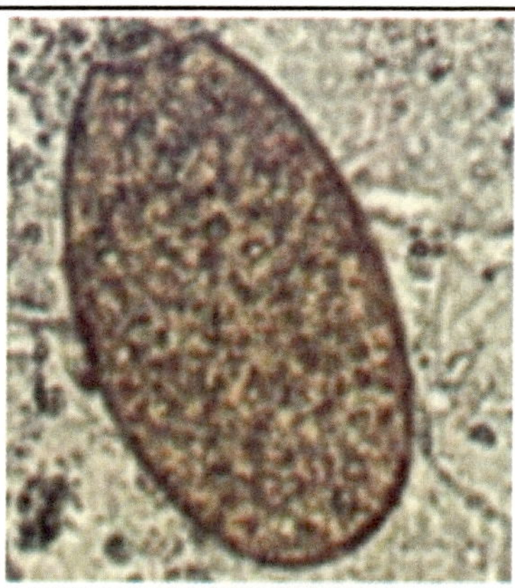

*Fasciola* sp.

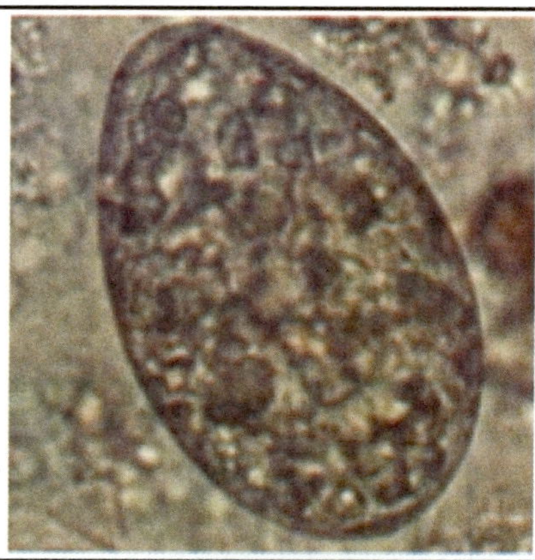

*Amphistome*

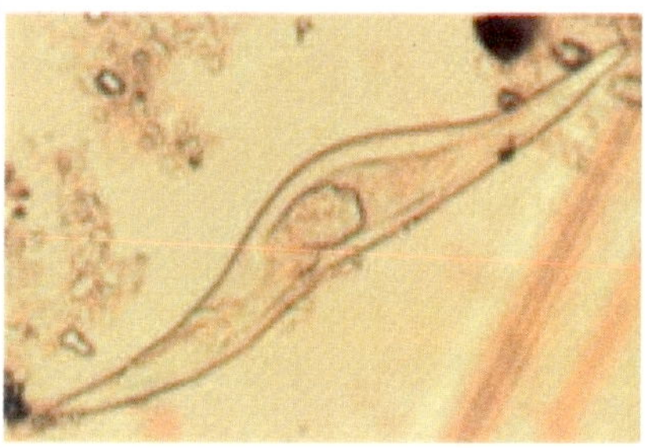

*Schistosoma nasale*

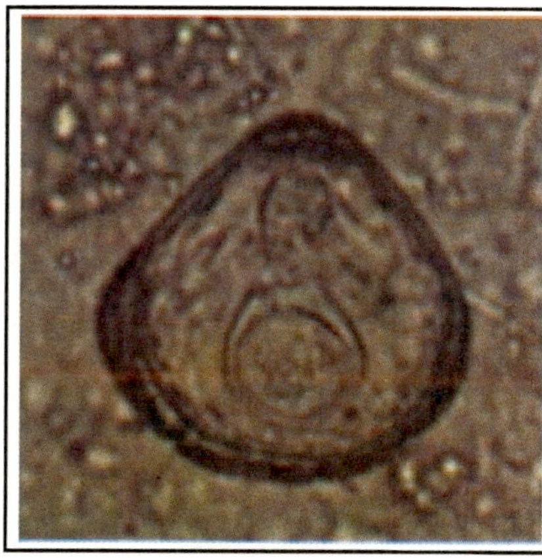

*Moniezia* sp.

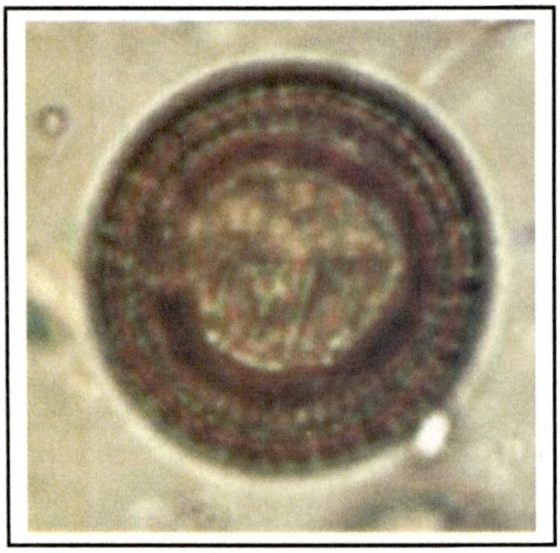

*Taenia* sp.

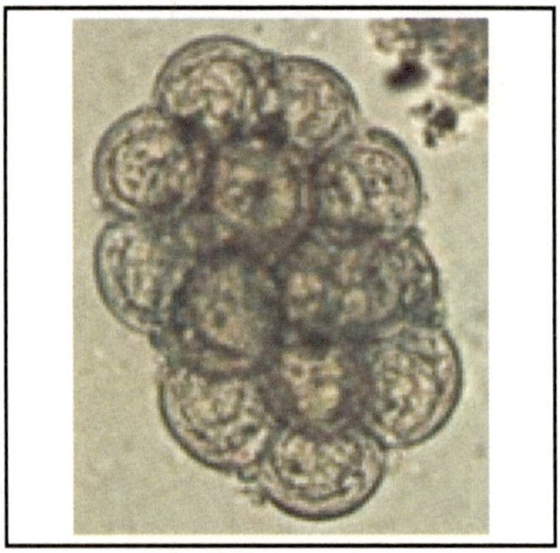

*Dipylidium caninum*

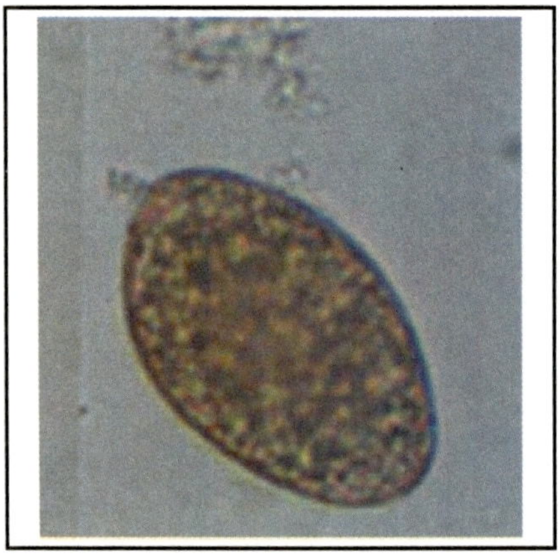

*Diphyllobothrium latum*

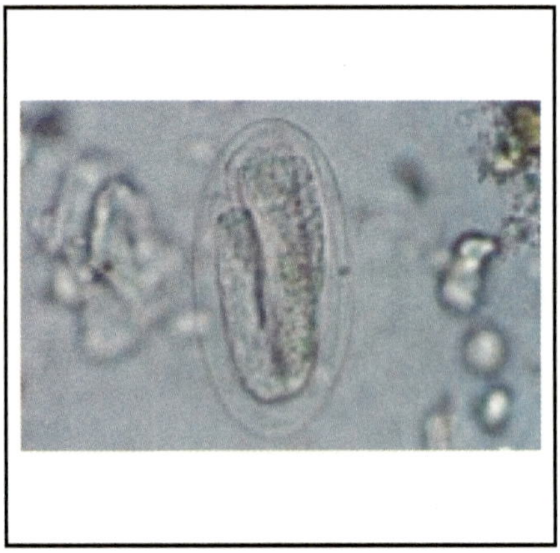

*Strongyloides* sp.

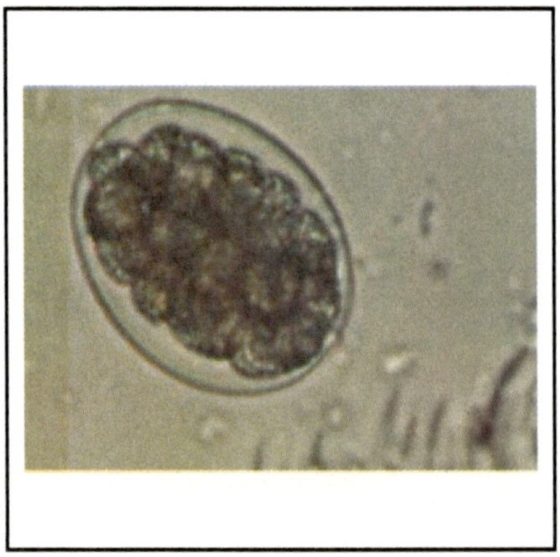

*Strongyle*

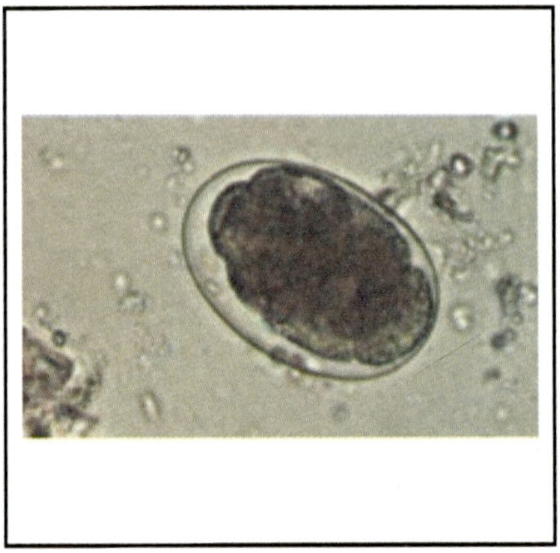

*Ancylostoma caninum*

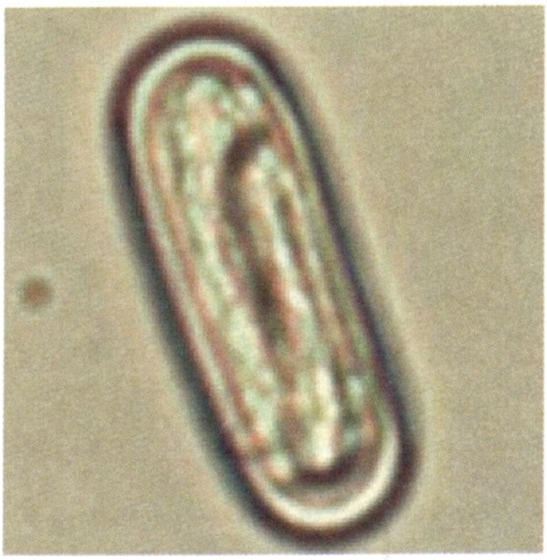

*Spirocerca lupi*

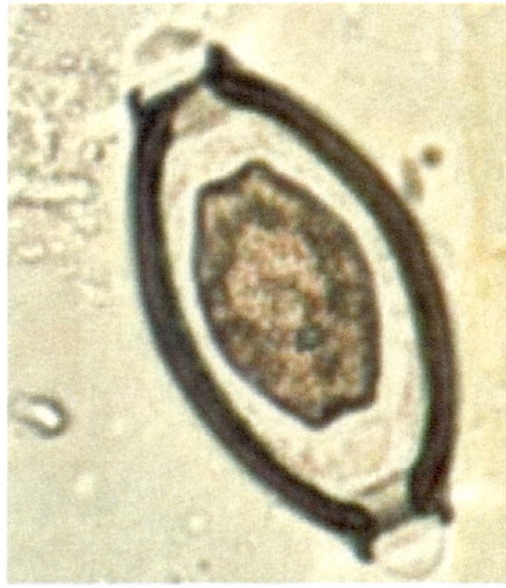

*Trichuris* sp.

## Annexure II: Wings of insects

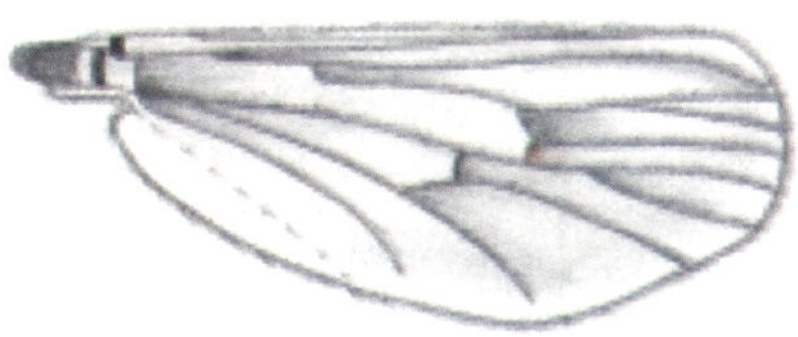

*Culicine mosquito*

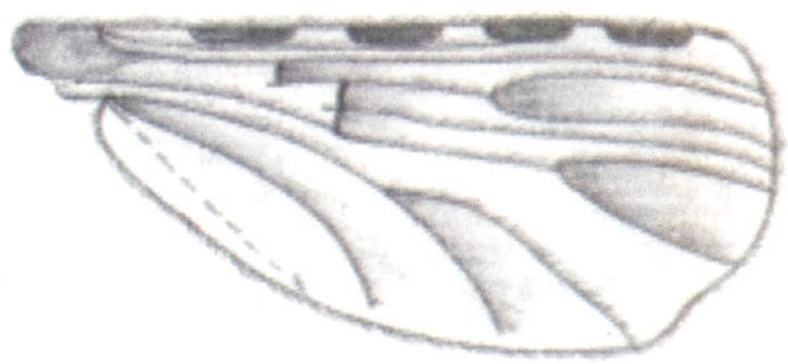

*Anopheline mosquito*

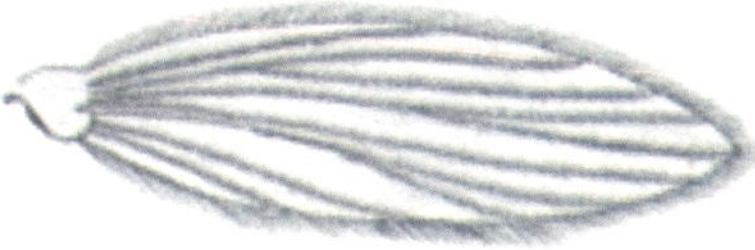

*Phlebotomus* sp.

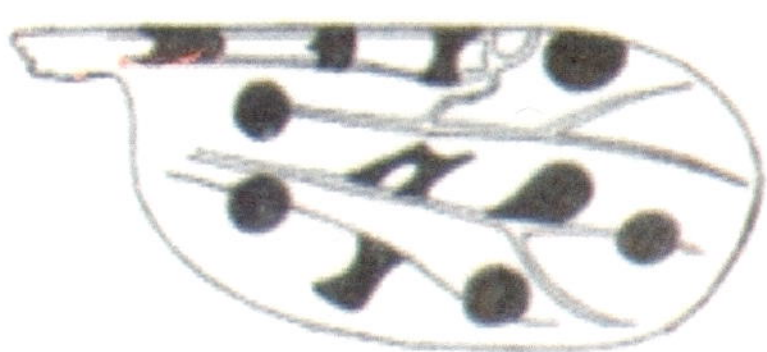

*Culicoides* sp.

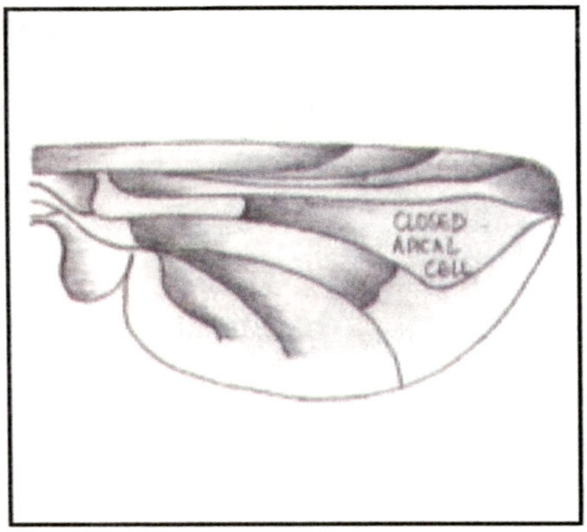


*Musca domestica*

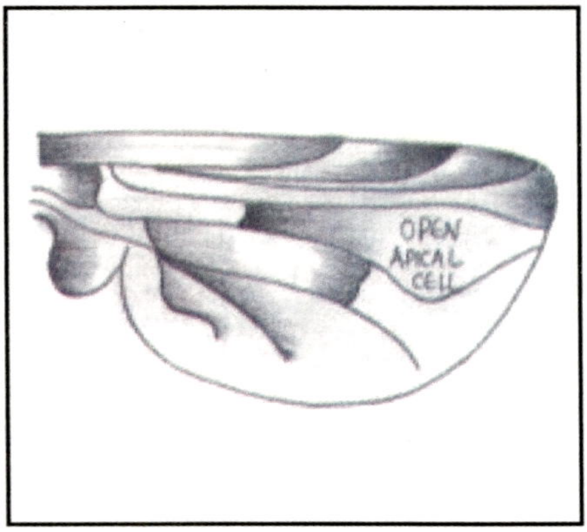


*Stomoxys calcitrans*

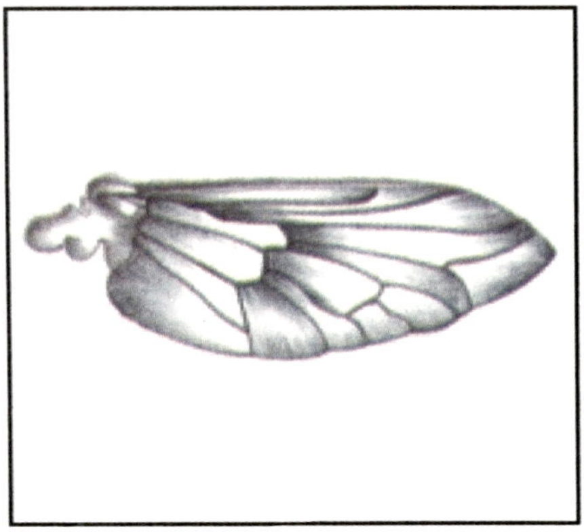

*Tabanus striatus*

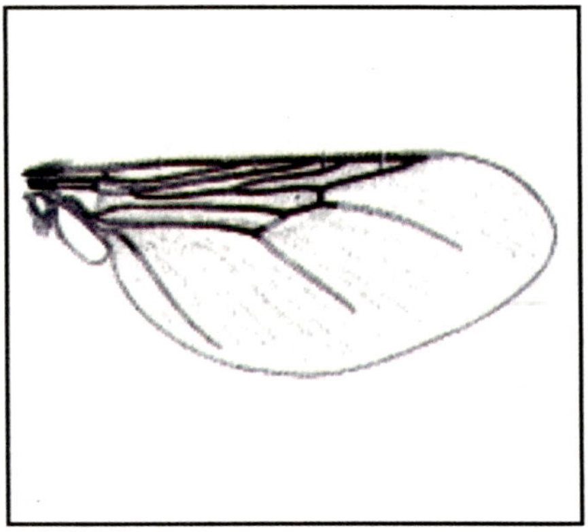

*Hippobosca maculata*

## Annexure III: Common Blood Protozoa

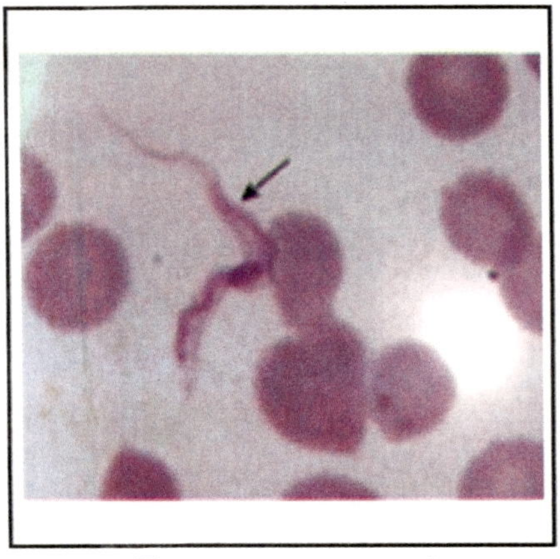

*Trypanosoma evansi*

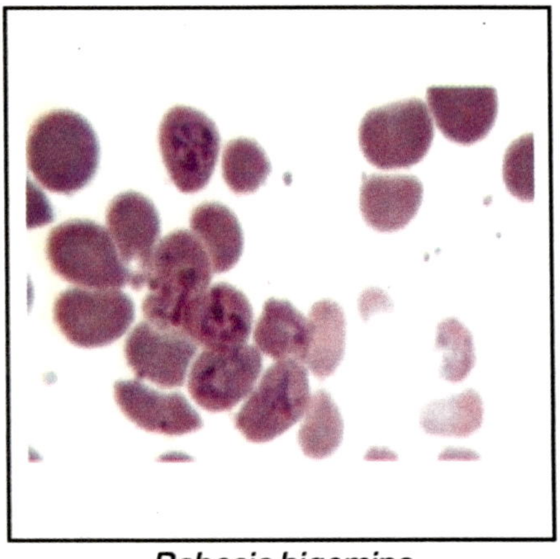

*Babesia bigemina*

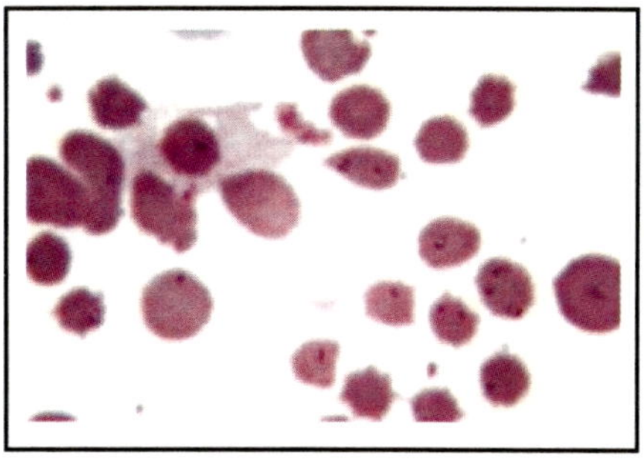

*Theileria annulata (Piroplasm)*

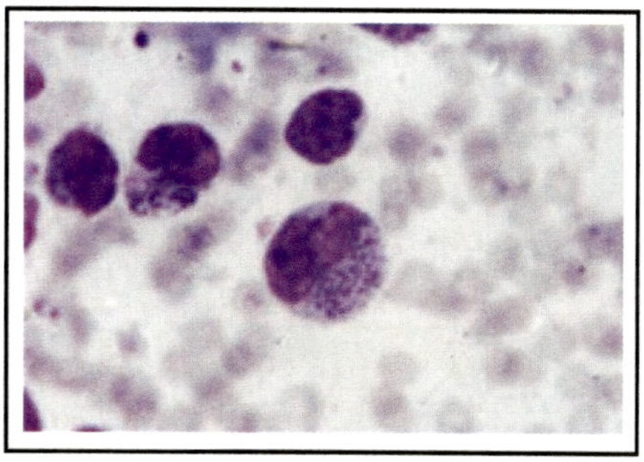

*Theileria annulata (Schizont or Koch's blue bodies)*

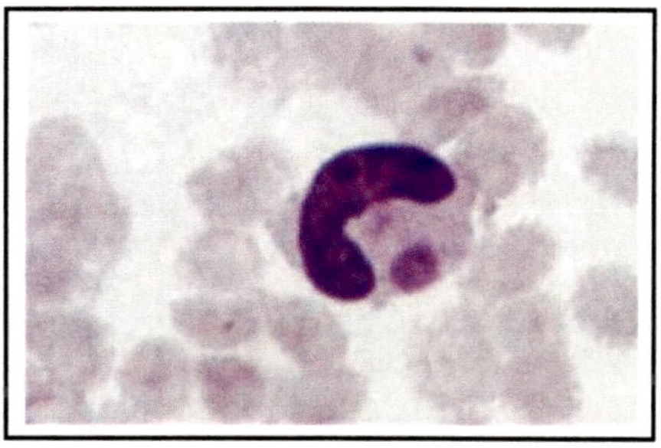

*Ehrlichia canis*

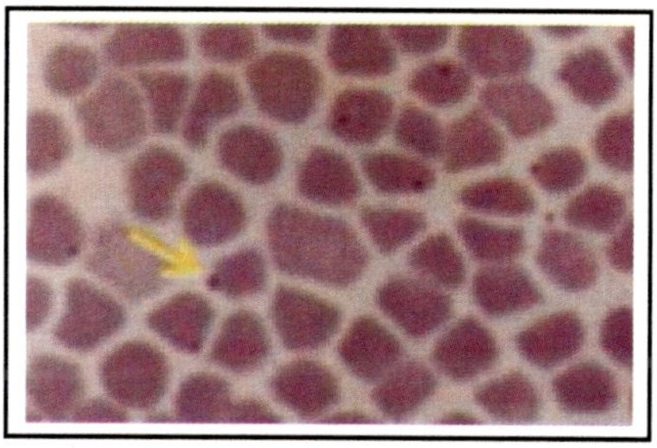

*Anaplasma marginale*

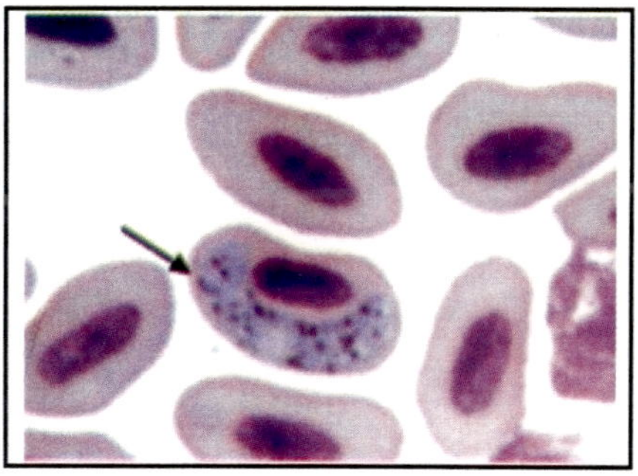

*Haemoproteus columbae*

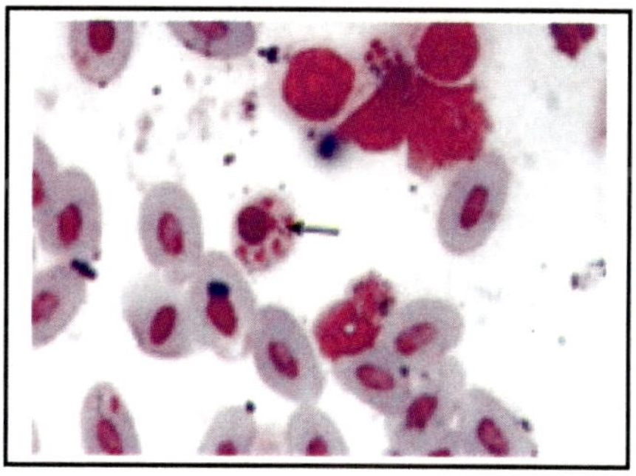

*Plasmodium gallinaceum*

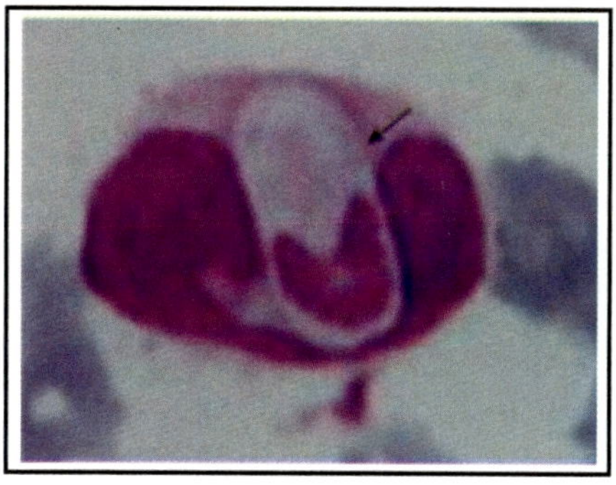

*Hepatozoon canis*

## ABOUT THE AUTHORS

**Dr. Bhaskaran Ravi Latha,** MVSc, Ph.D is currently the Professor and Head of the department of Veterinary Parasitology, Madras Veterinary College, Chennai having 24 years of experience in teaching Veterinary Parasitology to Undergraduate and Postgraduate students. She has guided several MVSc and Ph.D students and has done extensive research on ticks. She has worked as Principal Investigator and Co-Principal investigator in 13 research schemes. She is the recipient of the prestigious Tamil Nadu Scientists Award (TANSA award) in 2000 for her research work on the biology and bionomics of common ticks in Tamil Nadu. She has developed the e-module for Veterinary Entomology and Acarology course for Undergraduate Veterinary students. She is currently working on novel and ecofriendly pheromone based methods for tick control.

**Dr. S.T. Bino Sundar,** MVSc is currently working as Assistant Professor in the department of Veterinary Parasitology, Madras Veterinary College, Chennai. He did his under graduation from Veterinary College and Research Institute, Namakkal and post graduation from Veterinary College, Hebbal, Bangalore. He has been involved in teaching Veterinary Parasitology to Undergraduate Veterinary Students for 7 years. He also has 5 years of experience in the IT industry in the area of Knowledge process outsourcing where he was involved in projects related to pharmacology database development, journal excerption, patent analytics, medical key opinion leader profiling and clinical trial data management. He was also involved in using Information and Communication technologies (ICT) and resources for technology mediated learning process. He is currently working on the use of infochemical and herbal based methods in fly control.